CANCER ETIOLOGY, DIAGNOSIS AND TREATMENTS

AF761340

PATHOLOGICAL DIAGNOSIS OF BREAST CANCER

CANCER ETIOLOGY, DIAGNOSIS AND TREATMENTS

Additional books in this series can be found on Nova's website under the Series tab.

Additional e-books in this series can be found on Nova's website under the eBooks tab.

CANCER ETIOLOGY, DIAGNOSIS AND TREATMENTS

PATHOLOGICAL DIAGNOSIS OF BREAST CANCER

SACHIN B. INGLE
PRITI KATKADE
KUNDAN CHAVAN
AND
DATTA GIRJI

Nova Biomedical
New York

Library of Congress Cataloging-in-Publication Data

ISBN: 978-1-63485-171-8

Published by Nova Science Publishers, Inc. † New York

Contents

Preface

Breast tumors are one of the most worrisome and challenging problems for surgeons and pathologists. In this book, the authors present research in the study of the epidemiology, management and prevention of breast tumors; some examples of these types of breast cancer are DCIS, LCIS, IDC, ILC, medullary carcinoma, metaplastic carcinoma, papillary carcinoma, adenoid cystic carcinoma, and rare tumors of the breast. This book is definitely useful to surgeons and pathologists, postgraduates in understanding the pathology for diagnosis, treatment and prevention of these tumors.

Chapter 1 - Normal histology breast - Breast is a modified sweat gland. The breast or mammary gland is covered by skin and subcutaneous tissue and rests on the pectoralis muscle, from which it is separated by a fascia. In this chapter we will see about the normal histology of breast and the location of the tumor from which it arise. The normal ductular and lobular unit of the breast is studied.

Chapter 2 - Classification of the breast - Classification of the breast according to WHO criteria 2010 is studied in this chapter. It is very much important to categorize breast tumors for their prognostic and management point of view.

Chapter 3 - Etiopathogenesis of breast tumors - Breast carcinoma is the most common malignant tumor and the leading cause of carcinoma death in women, with more than 1 000 000 cases occurring worldwide annually. In the United States, approximately 100 000 new cases are diagnosed annually and approximately 30 000 patients die from the disease. The incidence is high in North America and northern Europe (91.4 new cases per 100 000 women/year), intermediate in southern European and Latin American countries, and low in most Asian and African countries (but rising rapidly in recent years with increased affluence of some of these countries). There are various modifiable and non modifiable risk factors in the development of breast tumors such as lifestyle changes, age at menarche, age at pregnancy, genetic factors etc,.

Chapter 4 - Ductal carcinoma in situ - DCIS is often detected with mammographies but can rarely be felt. With the increasing use of screening mammography, noninvasive cancers are more frequently diagnosed and now constitute 15% to 20% of all breast cancers. The specific causes of DCIS are still unknown. Women considered at higher risks are those who have a family history of breast cancer, those who have had their periods at an early age or who have had a late menopause. A lump or thickening in or near the breast or under the arm. A change in the size or shape of the breast. Nipple discharge or nipple tenderness; the nipple may also be inverted, or pulled back into the breast. On FNAC high grade DCIS shows large pleomorphic cells with malignant features in sheets, irregular aggregates and singles and low grade DCIS shows mild to moderate epithelial cells mainly cohesive, forming large sheets often with holes or papillary fragments. IHC positive for E-cadherin and scantiness or absence of HMW keratin.

Chapter 5 - Lobular carcinoma in situ - LCIS is usually diagnosed before menopause, most often between the ages of 40 & 50 years. Less than 10% of women diagnosed with LCIS have already gone through menopause. LCIS is extremely uncommon in men. Lobular carcinoma *in situ* (LCIS) is a condition caused by unusual cells in the lobules of the breast. Cells of LCIS and invasive lobular carcinoma have the same histology, appearing as single detached cells, as both have loss of expression of e-cadherin. Most of the risk relates to subsequent invasive ductal carcinoma rather than to invasive lobular carcinoma.

Chapter 6 - Invasive ductal carcinoma - Tumors included in this category are all those in which stromal invasion is detectable, whether an in situ component is identifiable or not, and regardless of the relative proportion of the two components. In other words, it also includes so-called 'microinvasive carcinoma.' Most commonly occurring in elderly women except secretory juvenile variant carcinoma which is seen in children. Patient presents with the lump in the breast most commonly involved quadrant is the upper outer quadrant, which is of increasing in size with short duration. In pagets disease it shows eczema of the nipple, in inflammatory carcinoma it shows inflammation and edema over the surface. Prognosis depends on the type of tumor and management is done on the basis of invasion shown by the tumor.

Chapter 7 - Invasive lobular carcinoma - Invasive lobular carcinoma accounts for 5-10% of invasive breast cancer. The grossly the tumor is fixed to the surrounding tissue with concave cut face. The tumor s hard, gritty ('unripe pear'), color is variable often streaked with yellow (elastic tissue). Characterized by presence of small and uniform tumor cells growing singly in Indian file pattern, concentric fashion around lobules.

Chapter 8 - Medullary carcinoma - Medullary carcinoma usually appears in patients under 50 years of age and is said to be particularly common in Japanese women. It is also said to be particularly common in carriers of *BRCA1* mutations. Grossly it is well circumscribed and may become large; it can be mistaken clinically and grossly for a fibroadenoma. The borders are always of the 'pushing' type. The pattern of growth is diffuse, with minimal or no glandular differentiation or intraductal growth and absence of mucin secretion. The prognosis for medullary carcinoma is better than for the ordinary invasive ductal carcinoma.

Chapter 9 - Metaplastic carcinoma - Heterogeneous group of neoplasms with predominant component other than epithelial/glandular. Uncommon (< 5% of breast carcinomas) More aggressive than invasive ductal NOS due to larger tumor size, higher grade Metastases tend to be hematogenous and not nodal. Grossly it is well-circumscribed.

Chapter 10 - Adenoid cystic carcinoma - Adenoid cystic carcinomas (ACCs) constitute 0.1–1% of all malignant breast tumors. They have better prognosis than other breast malignancies. To date, there have been about 933 cases reported as per English literature. It presents most commonly as a painful breast mass. In contrast to the aggressive nature of ACC at other sites, ACC of the breast has a favorable prognosis, lymph node involvement or distant metastases seldom occur. Treatment is basically of simple mastectomy. Chemotherapy, radiation and hormonal treatment have been infrequently used and evaluated.

Chapter 11 - Papillary carcinoma - Abstract - The term "intracystic papillary ductal carcinoma in situ" has recently been changed and is now more appropriately referred to as "intracystic papillary carcinoma'' constituting only 0.5% to 1% of all breast cancers. It is more frequently found among postmenopausal women with an average age between 55 and 67 years old. Intracystic (Encysted) papillary carcinoma (IPC) is a rare distinct entity with slow growth rate and overall favorable prognosis regardless of whether it is in situ alone or associated with invasive component. Treatment modalities vary from conservative surgery to radical surgery with or without adjuvant therapy depending upon the associated component (DCIS or invasive) of the tumor.

The oncosurgeon and oncopathologist should keep in mind this rare type of in situ carcinoma as a differential diagnosis in palpable breast lumps as it often mimics a benign lesion clinically. However, careful histopathological evaluation superadded by immunohistochemistry is an effective tool to arrive at the correct diagnosis to avoid untoward complications related to under diagnosis and/over diagnosis.

Chapter 12 - Rare tumors of the breast - Breast also shows some rare tumors such as angiosarcoma, adenoid cystic carcinoma, malignant lymphoma. Pathologists should also keep in mind about these rare tumors while reporting.

Chapter 1

Normal Histology of Breast

The breast or mammary gland is covered by skin and subcutaneous tissue and rests on the pectoralis muscle, from which it is separated by a fascia.

The morphofunctional unit of the organ is a single gland which is made up of two components Terminal Duct Lobular Unit (TDLU) and large duct system (Figure 1).

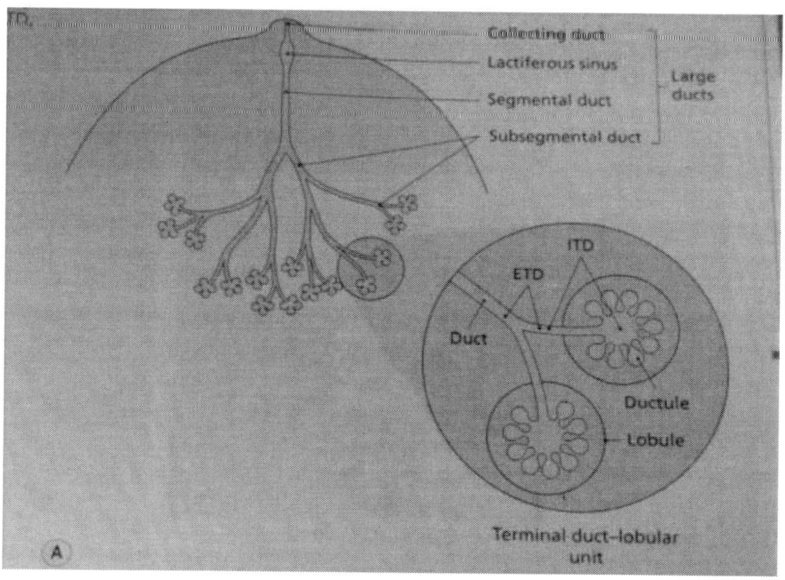

Figure 1. Showing TDLU and large duct.

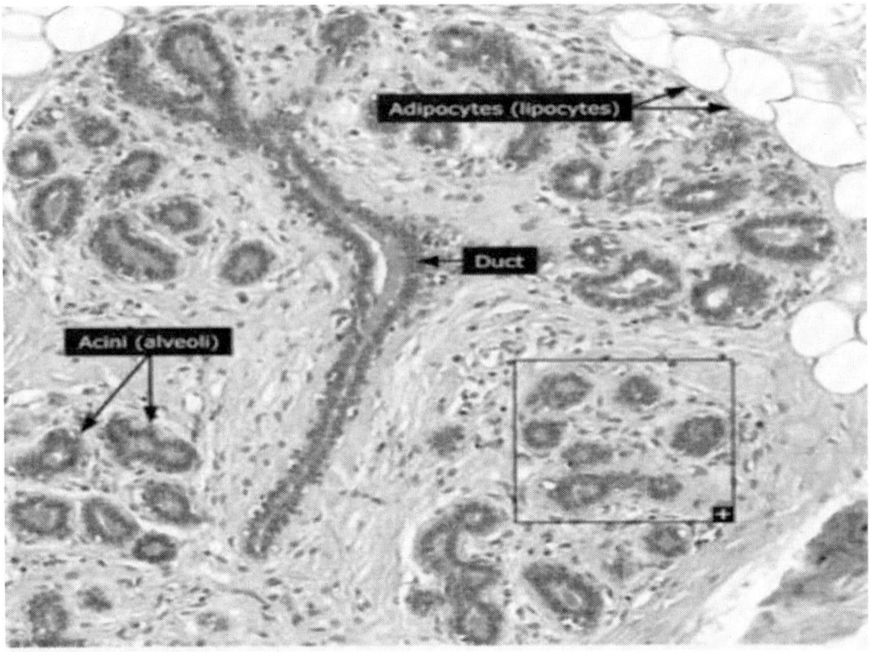

Figure 2. Showing normal histology of breast.

TDLU is mainly constituted by the lobule and terminal ductile. It represents the secretory portion of the gland. It connects with the subsegmental duct which in turn leads to segmental duct and this to a collecting duct which empties into the nipple. A fusiform dilation located beneath the nipple between the collecting and segmental duct is known as lactiferous sinus [1].

In adult women, the terminal duct branches into a grapelike cluster of small acini to form lobule [2]. The acini are surrounded by loose fibrovascular intralobular stroma which contrasts with the denser and less cellular interlobular stroma (Figure 2). Elastic tissue, normally present in variable amount around duct, is absent from the lobule.

The luminal epithelium of the resting breast is cuboidal or columnar. The outer basal or myoepithelial layer, although always present, is variably distinctive. In fresh tissue, myoepithelial cell can be demonstrated by staining for alkaline phosphatase activity, whereas in fixed tissue they can be demonstrated by IHC method [3].

The superficial portion are lined by keratinizing squamous cells that abruptly change to the double layered epithelium (luminal and myoepithelial cell) [2]. The epidermis of the nipple and areola resemble that of skin elsewhere, except for an increase in a melanin content in the basal layer and the occasional presence of basaly located clear cells known as Tokar cells which are related histogenetically to Paget disease.

Markers

The immunohistochemical Markers for epithelial cell include various keratins and EMA. Myoepithelial markers include S100, smooth musclc actin, calponin, P-cadherin, smooth muscle myosin, maspin and caldesmon [1].

Physiological Changes in Breast

In the prepubertal female breast and males, the large duct system ends in terminal ducts.

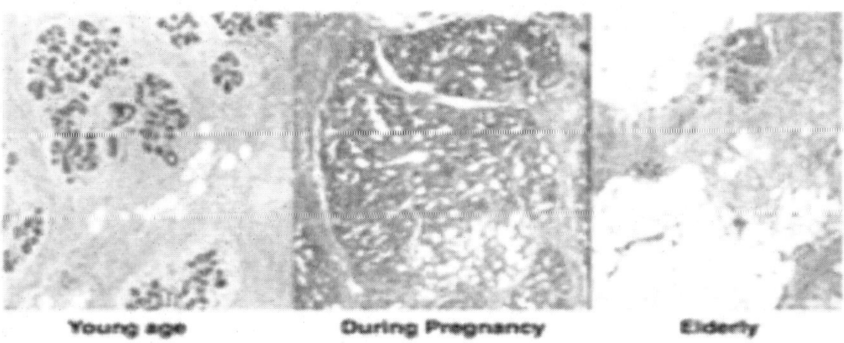

Figure 3. Showing physiological changes during various phases).

1) In the **first half of the menstrual cycle** the lobules are relatively quiescent.

2) **After ovulation** under the influence of estrogen and rising progesterone level, cell proliferation increases as does the number of acini per lobule. The intralobularstroma becomes markedly edematous.

3) **Upon menstruation the** fall in hormone levels induces the regression of the lobule and the disappearance of the edema.

4) In pregnancy lobules increase in number and size.

By the end of pregnancy breast is composed almost entirely by lobules separated by relatively scant stroma.

Immediately after parturition lobules produces colostrums, changing to milk over the next 10 days as the progesterone level drops.

5) **After the third decade long before menopause**, lobules and their specialized stroma start to involute and the interlobular stroma converts from radiodense fibrous stroma to radioluscent adipose tissue [2].

References

[1] Rosai Juan, Breast In: Rosai and Ackerman's surgical pathology Volume-2, 10th Ed. *Elsevier;* 2012; 1660-1661.

[2] Kumar V, Abbas AK, Aster JC, et al; Breast In: Robbins &Cotran Pathologic Basis of Disease Volume-2, South Asia Ed. *Elsevier;* 2014; 1043-104.

[3] Mills SE, Carter D, Greenson JK, Reuter VE, Stoler MH, et al; Breast In: Sternberg's Diagnostic Surgical Pathology Volume-1, 5th Ed. *Wolter Kluwer/Lippincott Williams & Wilkins; 2010*; 291-292.

Chapter 2

WHO Classification of Breast Tumors

The 2003 World Health Organization (WHO) classification of tumors of the breast [7] which includes benign (generally harmless) tumors and malignant (cancerous) tumors, recommends the following pathological types:

Invasive Breast Carcinomas

- Invasive ductal carcinoma
  - Most are "not otherwise specified"
  - The remainder are given subtypes:
    - Mixed type carcinoma
    - Pleomorphic carcinoma
    - Carcinoma with osteoclast giant cells
    - Carcinoma with choriocarcinoma features
    - Carcinoma with melanotic features
- Invasive lobular carcinoma
- Tubular carcinoma
- Invasive cribriform carcinoma
- Medullary carcinoma
- Mucinous carcinoma and other tumours with abundant mucin
  - Mucinous carcinoma

- Cystadenocarcinoma and columnar cell mucinous carcinoma
- Signet ring cell carcinoma
- Neuroendocrine tumours
    - Solid neuroendocrine carcinoma (carcinoid of the breast)
    - Atypical carcinoid tumor
    - Small cell/oat cell carcinoma
    - Large cell neuroendocrine carcinoma
- Invasive papillary carcinoma
- Invasive micropapillary carcinoma
- Apocrine carcinoma
- Metaplastic carcinomas
    - Pure epithelial metaplastic carcinomas
        - Squamous cell carcinoma
        - Adenocarcinoma with spindle cell metaplasia
        - Adenosquamous carcinoma
        - Mucoepidermoid carcinoma
    - Mixed epithelial/mesenchymal metaplastic carcinomas

(Other well-accepted subtypes of metaplastic mammary carcinoma thought to have clinical significance but not included in the decade old WHO classification:

- Matrix-producing carcinoma
- Spindle cell carcinoma
- Carcinosarcoma
- Squamous cell carcinoma of mammary origin
- Metaplastic carcinoma with osteoclastic giant cells)

- Lipid-rich carcinoma
- Secretory carcinoma
- Oncocytic carcinoma
- Adenoid cystic carcinoma
- Acinic cell carcinoma
- Glycogen-rich clear cell carcinoma
- Sebaceous carcinoma
- Inflammatory carcinoma
- Bilateral breast carcinoma

Mesenchymal Tumors (Including Sarcoma)

- Hemangioma
- Angiomatosis
- Hemangiopericytoma
- Pseudoangiomatous stromal hyperplasia
- Myofibroblastoma
- Fibromatosis (aggressive)
- Inflammatory myofibroblastic tumor
- Lipoma
    - Angiolipoma
- Granular cell tumour
- Neurofibroma
- Schwannoma
- Angiosarcoma
- Liposarcoma
- Rhabdomyosarcoma
- Osteosarcoma
- Leiomyoma
- Leiomyosarcoma

Tumors of the Male Breast

- Gynecomastia (benign)
- Carcinoma
    - In situ
    - Invasive

Malignant Lymphoma

- Non-Hodgkin lymphoma

Metastatic tumors to the breast from other places in the body

Precursor Lesions

- Lobular neoplasia
    - lobular carcinoma in situ
- Intraductal proliferative lesions
    - Usual ductal hyperplasia
    - Flat epithelial hyperplasia
    - Atypical ductal hyperplasia
    - Ductal carcinoma in situ
- Microinvasive carcinoma
- Intraductal papillary neoplasms
    - Central papilloma
    - Peripheral papilloma
    - Atypical papilloma
    - Intraductal papillary carcinoma
    - Intracystic papillary carcinoma

Benign Epithelial Lesions

- Adenosis, including variants
    - Sclerosing adenosis
    - Apocrine adenosis
    - Blunt duct adenosis
    - Microglandular adenosis
    - Adenomyoepithelial adenosis
- Radial scar/complex sclerosing lesion
- Adenomas
    - Tubular adenoma
    - Lactating adenoma
    - Apocrine adenoma
    - Pleomorphic adenoma
    - Ductal adenoma

Myoepithelial Lesions

- Myoepitheliosis
- Adenomyoepithelial adenosis
- Adenomyoepithelioma
- Malignant myoepithelioma

Fibroepithelial Tumours

- Fibroadenoma
- Phyllodes tumour
  - Benign
  - Borderline
  - Malignant
- Periductal stromal sarcoma, low-grade
- Mammary hamartoma

Benign Tumors of the Nipple

- Nipple adenoma
- Syringomatous adenoma
- Paget's disease of the nipple

Malignant Tumors of the Nipple

- Paget's disease of the nipple

References

[1] Gonzalez-Angulo AM, Morales-Vasquez F, Hortobagyi GN (2007). "Overview of resistance to systemic therapy in patients with breast cancer." *Adv. Exp. Med. Biol. Advances in Experimental Medicine and*

Biology 608: 1–22. doi:10.1007/978-0-387-74039-3_1. ISBN 978-0-387-74037-9. PMID 17993229.

[2] Giordano SH, Hortobagyi GN (2003). "Inflammatory breast cancer: Clinical progress and the main problems that must be addressed." *Breast Cancer Res.* 5 (6): 284–8. doi:10.1186/bcr608. PMC 314400. PMID 14580242.

[3] Merck Manual, Professional Edition, Ch. 253, *Breast Cancer.*

[4] Percentage values are from United States statistics 2004. Subtype specific incidences are taken from Table 6 (invasive) and Table 3 (in situ) from Eheman CR, Shaw KM, Ryerson AB, Miller JW, Ajani UA, White MC (June 2009). "The changing incidence of in situ and invasive ductal and lobular breast carcinomas: United States, 1999–2004." Cancer Epidemiol. Biomarkers Prev. 18 (6): 1763–9. doi:10.1158/1055-9965. EPI-08-1082. PMID 19454615. These are divided by total breast cancer incidence (211,300 invasive and 55,700 in situ cases) as reported from Breast Cancer Facts & Figures 2003–2004 [1] [dead link].

[5] NOTE: Number really refers to invasive ductal carcinoma, despite title. Arpino G, Bardou VJ, Clark GM, Elledge RM (2004). "Infiltrating lobular carcinoma of the breast: tumor characteristics and clinical outcome." *Breast Cancer Res.* 6 (3): R149–56. doi:10.1186/bcr767. PMC 400666. PMID 15084238.

[6] Evans, A. (2004). "Ductal carcinoma in situ (DCIS): are we overdetecting it?". *Breast Cancer Research* 6: P23. doi:10.1186/bcr842. [2].

[7] World Health Organization: Tumours of the Breast and Female Genital Organs. Oxford [Oxfordshire]: *Oxford University Press*. 2003. ISBN 92-832-2412-4.

[8] Elston CW, Ellis IO. Pathologic prognostic factors in breast cancer. I. The value of histological grades in breast cancer. Experience from a large study with long-term follow-up. *Histopathology* 1991, 19:403-410.

[9] Bloom, H.J.; Richardson, W.W. (1957). "Histological grading and prognosis in breast cancer; A study of 1409 cases of which 359 have been followed for 15 years." *British Journal of Cancer* 11 (3): 359–77. doi:10.1038/bjc.1957.43. PMC 2073885. PMID 13499785.

[10] Genestie, C.; Zafrani, B.; Asselain, B.; Fourquet, A.; Rozan, S.; Validire, P.; Vincent-Salomon, A.; Sastre-Garau, X. (1998). "Comparison of the prognostic value of Scarff-Bloom-Richardson and Nottingham histological grades in a series of 825 cases of breast cancer: Major

importance of the mitotic count as a component of both grading systems." *Anticancer Research* 18 (1B): 571–6. PMID 9568179.
[11] National Comprehensive Cancer Network (NCCN) guidelines, Breast Cancer Version 2.2011 http://www.nccn.org/professionals/physician_gls/pdf/breast.pdf.
[12] What is Cancer Staging? American Joint Committee on Cancer 2010 May 5.http://www.cancerstaging.org/mission/whatis.html.
[13] National Cancer Institute. Stage Information for Breast Cancer.http://www.cancer.gov/cancertopics/pdq/treatment/breast/healthprofessional/page3.
[14] American Joint Committee on Cancer. Past Editions of the AJCC Cancer Staging Manual available at http://www.cancerstaging.org/products/pasteditions.html.
[15] AJCC Cancer Staging Manual, 7th edition, updated Cancer Staging Posters.http://www.cancerstaging.org/staging/posters/breast8.5x11.pdf.
[16] AJCC Cancer Staging Manual 6th edition; Chapter 25; Breast Cancer – original pages 223-240 http://www.cancerstaging.org/products/csmanual6ed-4.pdf.
[17] AJCC Cancer Staging Manual 5th edition; Chapter 25; Breast Cancer – original pages 171-180 http://www.cancerstaging.org/products/csmanual5ed_4.pdf.
[18] AJCC Cancer Staging Manual 4th edition; Chapter 25; Breast Cancer – original pages 149-154 http://www.cancerstaging.org/products/csmanual4ed_2.pdf.
[19] AJCC Cancer Staging Manual 3rd edition; 1988; Chapter 23; Breast Cancer-original pages 145-150 http://www.cancerstaging.org/products/csmanual3ed_2.pdf.
[20] AJCC Cancer Staging Manual 2nd edition; 1983; Chapter 21; Breast Cancer-original pages 127-134 http://www.cancerstaging.org/products/csmanual2ed.pdf.
[21] AJCC Cancer Staging Manual 1977; Chapter 12; Breast Cancer-original pages 101-108 http://www.cancerstaging.org/products/csmanual1ed.pdf.
[22] Feinstein, A. R.; Sosin, D. M.; Wells, C. K. (1985). "The Will Rogers Phenomenon." *New England Journal of Medicine* 312 (25): 1604–1608. doi:10.1056/NEJM198506203122504. PMID 4000199.
[23] Woodward, W. A.; Strom, E. A.; Tucker, S. L.; McNeese, M. D.; Perkins, G. H.; Schechter, N. R.; Singletary, S. E.; Theriault, R. L.; Hortobagyi, G. N.; Hunt, K. K.; Buchholz, T. A. (2003). "Changes in the 2003 American Joint Committee on Cancer Staging for Breast Cancer

Dramatically Affect Stage-Specific Survival." *Journal of Clinical Oncology* 21 (17): 3244–3248. doi:10.1200/JCO.2003.03.052. PMID 12947058.

[24] Scatarige JC, Fishman EK, Zinreich ES, Brem RF, Almaraz R (April 1988). "Internal mammary lymphadenopathy in breast carcinoma: CT appraisal of anatomic distribution." *Radiology* 167 (1): 89–91. doi:10.1148/radiology.167.1.3347753. PMID 3347753.

[25] Scatarige JC, Boxen I, Smathers RL (September 1990). "Internal mammary lymphadenopathy: imaging of a vital lymphatic pathway in breast cancer." Radiographics 10 (5): 857–70. doi:10.1148/radiographics.10.5.2217975. PMID 2217975. available as full text article with multiple images at http://radiographics.rsna.org/content/10/5/857.full.pdf.

[26] Kumar, V; Abbas, AK; Fausto, N; Mitchell, R. "19 – The Female Genital System and Breast." *Robbins Basic Pathology*. (8th ed.). p. 749. ISBN 1416029737.

[27] Molecular origin of cancer: gene-expression signatures in breast cancer, Christos Sotirou and Lajos Pusztai, *N Engl J Med* 360:790 (2009 Feb 19).

[28] Romond EH, Perez EA, Bryant J, et al. Trastuzumab plus adjuvant chemotherapy for operable HER2+ breast cancer. *N Engl J Med.* 2005; 353:1673-1684 and supplementary appendix.

[29] Dent R, Trudeau M, Pritchard KI, Hanna WM, Kahn HK; et al. (2007-08-01). "Triple-Negative Breast Cancer: Clinical Features and Patterns of Recurrence." Clinical Cancer Research (American Association for Cancer Research) 13 (15 Pt 1): 4429–4434. doi:10.1158/1078-0432.CCR-06-3045. PMID 17671126.

[30] "Understanding and Treating Triple-Negative Breast Cancer." Cancer Network. Retrieved 2010-05-08.

[31] Lehmann, B. D.; Bauer, J. A.; Chen, X.; Sanders, M. E.; Chakravarthy, A. B.; Shyr, Y.; Pietenpol, J. A. (2011). "Identification of human triple-negative breast cancer subtypes and preclinical models for selection of targeted therapies." *Journal of Clinical Investigation* 121 (7): 2750–2767. doi:10.1172/JCI45014. PMC 3127435. PMID 21633166.

[32] Hu, R.; Dawood, S.; Holmes, M. D.; Collins, L. C.; Schnitt, S. J.; Cole, K.; Marotti, J. D.; Hankinson, S. E.; Colditz, G. A.; Tamimi, R. M. (2011). "Androgen Receptor Expression and Breast Cancer Survival in Postmenopausal Women." *Clinical Cancer Research* 17 (7): 1867–1874. doi:10.1158/1078-0432.CCR-10-2021. PMC 3076683. PMID 21325075.

[33] Prat, A.; Perou, C. M. (2011). "Deconstructing the molecular portraits of breast cancer." *Molecular Oncology* 5 (1): 5–23. doi:10.1016/j.molonc. 2010.11.003. PMID 21147047.

[34] Geyer, F. C.; Marchiò, C.; Reis-Filho, J. S. (2009). "The role of molecular analysis in breast cancer." *Pathology* 41 (1): 77–88. doi:10.1080/00313020802563536. PMID 19089743.

[35] Perou, C. M. (2011). "Molecular Stratification of Triple-Negative Breast Cancers." *The Oncologist* 16: 61–70. doi:10.1634/theoncologist.2011-S1-61.

[36] Ross, J. S. (2009). "Multigene Classifiers, Prognostic Factors, and Predictors of Breast Cancer Clinical Outcome." *Advances in Anatomic Pathology* 16 (4): 204–215. doi:10.1097/PAP.0b013e3181a9d4bf. PMID 19546609.

[37] Herschkowitz, J. I.; Zhao, W.; Zhang, M.; Usary, J.; Murrow, G.; Edwards, D.; Knezevic, J.; Greene, S. B.; Darr, D.; Troester, M. A.; Hilsenbeck, S. G.; Medina, D.; Perou, C. M.; Rosen, J. M. (2011). "Breast Cancer Special Feature: Comparative oncogenomics identifies breast tumors enriched in functional tumor-initiating cells." *Proceedings of the National Academy of Sciences* 109 (8): 2778. doi:10.1073/pnas. 1018862108.

[38] Harrell, J. C.; Prat, A.; Parker, J. S.; Fan, C.; He, X.; Carey, L.; Anders, C.; Ewend, M.; Perou, C. M. (2011). "Genomic analysis identifies unique signatures predictive of brain, lung, and liver relapse." *Breast Cancer Research and Treatment* 132 (2): 523–535. doi:10.1007/s10549-011-1619-7. PMC 3303043. PMID 21671017.

[39] Perou CM, Sørlie T, Eisen MB; et al. (August 2000). "Molecular portraits of human breast tumours." *Nature* 406 (6797): 747–52. doi:10.1038/35021093. PMID 10963602.

[40] Nagasaki K, Miki Y (2006). "Gene expression profiling of breast cancer." *Breast Cancer* 13 (1): 2–7. doi:10.2325/jbcs.13.2. PMID 16518 056.

[41] Normanno N, De Luca A, Carotenuto P, Lamura L, Oliva I, D'Alessio A (2009). "Prognostic applications of gene expression signatures in breast cancer." Oncology. 77 Suppl 1: 2–8. doi:10.1159/000258489. PMID 20130425.

[42] Jönsson G, Staaf J, Vallon-Christersson J; et al. (2010). "Genomic subtypes of breast cancer identified by array-comparative genomic hybridization display distinct molecular and clinical characteristics."

Breast Cancer Res. 12 (3): R42. doi:10.1186/bcr2596. PMC 2917037. PMID 20576095.

[43] Sparano JA, Solin LJ (April 2010). "Defining the clinical utility of gene expression assays in breast cancer: the intersection of science and art in clinical decision making." *J. Clin. Oncol.* 28 (10): 1625–7. doi:10.1200/JCO.2009.25.2882. PMID 20065178.

[44] Mandrekar SJ, Sargent DJ (October 2010). "Predictive biomarker validation in practice: lessons from real trials." *Clin Trials* 7 (5): 567–73. doi:10.1177/1740774510368574. PMID 20392785.

[45] Pharoah PD, Caldas C (November 2010). "Genetics: How to validate a breast cancer prognostic signature." *Nat Rev Clin Oncol* 7 (11): 615–6. doi:10.1038/nrclinonc.2010.142. PMID 20981123.

[46] Ross, J. S.; Hatzis, C.; Symmans, W. F.; Pusztai, L.; Hortobagyi, G. N. (2008). "Commercialized Multigene Predictors of Clinical Outcome for Breast Cancer." *The Oncologist* 13 (5): 477–493. doi:10.1634/theoncologist.2007-0248. PMID 18515733.

[47] Albain, K. S.; Paik, S.; Van't Veer, L. (2009). "Prediction of adjuvant chemotherapy benefit in endocrine responsive, early breast cancer using multigene assays." *The Breast* 18: S141–S145. doi:10.1016/S0960-9776(09)70290-5. PMID 19914534.

[48] Fan, C.; Oh, D. S.; Wessels, L.; Weigelt, B.; Nuyten, D. S. A.; Nobel, A. B.; Van't Veer, L. J.; Perou, C. M. (2006). "Concordance among Gene-Expression–Based Predictors for Breast Cancer." *New England Journal of Medicine* 355 (6): 560–569. doi:10.1056/NEJMoa052933. PMID 16899776.

[49] Harris, L.; Fritsche, H.; Mennel, R.; Norton, L.; Ravdin, P.; Taube, S.; Somerfield, M. R.; Hayes, D. F.; Bast Jr, R. C.; American Society of Clinical Oncology (2007). "American Society of Clinical Oncology 2007 Update of Recommendations for the Use of Tumor Markers in Breast Cancer." *Journal of Clinical Oncology* 25 (33): 5287–5312. doi:10.1200/JCO.2007.14.2364. PMID 17954709.

[50] Armen Hareyanon. MapQuant Dx Genomic Grade Test Identifies Breast Cancer Patients. 2008-06-02 http://www.emaxhealth.com/98/22731.html.

[51] Filho, O. M.; Ignatiadis, M.; Sotiriou, C. (2011). "Genomic Grade Index: An important tool for assessing breast cancer tumor grade and prognosis." *Critical Reviews in Oncology/Hematology* 77 (1): 20–29. doi:10.1016/j.critrevonc.2010.01.011. PMID 20138540.

[52] "Select your country: Qiagen Marseille" (PDF). ipsogen.com. Retrieved 12 December 2015.[dead link].

[53] Gianni L, Zambetti M, Clark K; et al. (October 2005). "Gene expression profiles in paraffin-embedded core biopsy tissue predict response to chemotherapy in women with locally advanced breast cancer." *J. Clin. Oncol.* 23 (29): 7265–77. doi:10.1200/JCO.2005.02.0818. PMID 16145055.

[54] Kelly CM, Krishnamurthy S, Bianchini G; et al. (November 2010). "Utility of oncotype DX risk estimates in clinically intermediate risk hormone receptor-positive, HER2-normal, grade II, lymph node-negative breast cancers." *Cancer* 116 (22): 5161–7. doi:10.1002/cncr. 25269. PMID 20665886.

[55] Lo, S. S.; Mumby, P. B.; Norton, J.; Rychlik, K.; Smerage, J.; Kash, J.; Chew, H. K.; Gaynor, E. R.; Hayes, D. F.; Epstein, A.; Albain, K. S. (2010). "Prospective Multicenter Study of the Impact of the 21-Gene Recurrence Score Assay on Medical Oncologist and Patient Adjuvant Breast Cancer Treatment Selection." *Journal of Clinical Oncology* 28 (10): 1671–1676. doi:10.1200/JCO.2008.20.2119. PMID 20065191.

[56] Albanell, J.; González, A.; Ruiz-Borrego, M.; Alba, E.; García-Saenz, J. A.; Corominas, J. M.; Burgues, O.; Furio, V.; Rojo, A.; Palacios, J.; Bermejo, B.; Martínez-García, M.; Limon, M. L.; Muñoz, A. S.; Martín, M.; Tusquets, I.; Rojo, F.; Colomer, R.; Faull, I.; Lluch, A. (2011). "Prospective transGEICAM study of the impact of the 21-gene Recurrence Score assay and traditional clinicopathological factors on adjuvant clinical decision making in women with estrogen receptor-positive (ER+) node-negative breast cancer." *Annals of Oncology* 23 (3): 625–631. doi:10.1093/annonc/mdr278. PMID 21652577.

[57] New Mexico OncologyHematology Consultants, Ltd. Copyright held by CancerConsultants Breast Cancer Information Center. European Study Reports that Oncotype DX Influences Breast Cancer Treatment Decisions. Posted 2010 October 17, accessioned 2010 Dec 19 and 2011 July 03 at http://nmcancercenter.org/european-study-reports-that-oncotype-dx%C2%AE-influences-breast-cancer-treatment-decisions/.

[58] Tice JA. The 70-Gene Signature (MammaPrint) as a Guide for the Management of Early Stage Breast Cancer. California Technology Assessment Forum. 2010 June 2nd. Full text accessioned 2010 Dec 19 at http://www.ctaf.org/content/assessments/detail/?id=1178.

[59] NCI Cancer Bulletin FDA Update 2007 February 14, Volume 4, Number 7 as retrieved 2010 October 17 at http://www.cancer.gov/aboutnci/ncicancerbulletin/archive/2007/021407/page5.

[60] The mission of Agendia. Agendia web site.http://www.agendia.com/pages/mission/86.php.

[61] Ordering Symphony is a simple process. Agendia web site.http://www.agendia.com/pages/ordering_symphony/38.php.

[62] MammaPrint Patient Eligibility Internationally (Outside of the USA) http://www.agendia.com/pages/patient_eligibility_internationally/317.php.

[63] Introducing BluePrint: A Molecular Subtyping Profile for Breast Cancer. Agendia web site.http://www.agendia.com/pages/blueprint/324.php.

[64] DNA topoisomerase II alfa expression and the response to primary chemotherapy in breast cancer. MacGrogan G et al. *British Journal of Cancer* 2003; 89: 666–671. doi:10.1038/sj.bjc.6601185 www.bjcancer.com.

[65] Gene Review TOP2A – topoisomerase (DNA) II alpha 170kDa Homo sapiens as retrieved 2010 October 18 http://www.wikigenes.org/e/gene/e/7153.html.

[66] Alvarez, R. H.; Valero, V.; Hortobagyi, G. N. (2010). "Emerging Targeted Therapies for Breast Cancer." *Journal of Clinical Oncology* 28 (20): 3366–3379. doi:10.1200/JCO.2009.25.4011. PMID 20530283.

[67] Tutt A *J Clin Onc* 2009; 27(suppl 15): abst CRA501.

[68] Issaeva N, Thomas HD, Djureinovic T; et al. (August 2010). "6-thioguanine selectively kills BRCA2 defective tumours and overcomes PARP inhibitor resistance." *Cancer Res.* 70 (15): 6268–76. doi:10.1158/0008-5472.CAN-09-3416.PMC 2913123.PMID 206310 63.Correction published at Correction: 6-Thioguanine Selectively Kills BRCA2-Defective Tumors and Overcomes PARP Inhibitor Resistance *Cancer Res* 2010 October 1;70:7734.

[69] Baselga J et al. *J Clin Oncol* 2009; 27: 2630–2637.

[70] D'Anello L, Sansone P, Storci G; et al. (2010). "Epigenetic control of the basal-like gene expression profile via Interleukin-6 in breast cancer cells." *Mol. Cancer* 9: 300. doi:10.1186/1476-4598-9-300. PMC 3002335. PMID 21092249.

[71] Liu, C. -C.; Prior, J.; Piwnica-Worms, D.; Bu, G. (2010). "LRP6 overexpression defines a class of breast cancer subtype and is a target for therapy." *Proceedings of the National Academy of Sciences* 107 (11):

5136–5141. doi:10.1073/pnas.0911220107. PMC 2841938. PMID 2019 4742.

[72] Rae JM, Drury S, Hayes DF et al. Lack of Correlation between Gene Variants in Tamoxifen Metabolizing Enymes with Primary Endpoints in the ATAC Trial. 33rd Annual San Antonio Breast Cancer Symposium (SABCS): abstract S1-7 presented 2010 December 9; accessioned 2010 December 17 at http://www.abstracts2view.com/sabcs10/view.php?nu=SABCS10L_1093&terms=.

[73] Leyland-Jones B, Regan MM, Bouzyk M et al. Outcome According to CYP2D6 Genotype among Postmenopausal Women with Endocrine-Responsive Early Invasive Breast Cancer Randomized in the BIG 1-98 Trial. 33rd Annual San Antonio Breast Cancer Symposium (SABCS): abstract S1-8 presented 2010, December 9; accessioned 2010 December 17 at http://www.abstracts2view.com/sabcs10/view.php?nu=SABCS10L_556&terms=.

[74] Ruiter R; Bijl MJ; van Schaik RHN et al. CYP2C19*2 Polymorphism is Associated with Increased Survival in Breast Cancer Patients Using Tamoxifen. *Pharmacogenomics.* 2010;11(10):1367–1375.

[75] Jerevall P; Jansson A; Fornander T et al. Predictive Relevance of HOXB13 Protein Expression for Tamoxifen Benefit in Breast Cancer. *Breast Cancer Research.* 2010;12(206).

[76] "Study sheds new light on tamoxifen resistance." CORDIS: News. 2008-11-13. Hurtado A, Holmes KA, Geistlinger TR; et al. (December 2008). "ERBB2 regulation by Estrogen Receptor-Pax2 determines tamoxifen response." *Nature* 456 (7222): 663–6. doi:10.1038/nature 07483. PMC 2920208. PMID 19005469.

[77] Mc Ilroy M, Fleming FJ, Buggy Y, Hill AD, Young LS (December 2006). "Tamoxifen-induced ER-alpha-SRC-3 interaction in HER2 positive human breast cancer; a possible mechanism for ER isoform specific recurrence." *Endocr. Relat. Cancer* 13 (4): 1135–45. doi:10.1677/erc.1.01222. PMID 17158759.

[78] Spears M, Bartlett J (June 2009). "The potential role of estrogen receptors and the SRC family as targets for the treatment of breast cancer." *Expert Opin. Ther. Targets* 13 (6): 665–74. doi:10.1517/1472 8220902911509. PMID 19456271.

[79] [3][dead link].

[80] Ravdin PM, Siminoff LA, Davis GJ; et al. (February 2001). "Computer program to assist in making decisions about adjuvant therapy for women

with early breast cancer." *J. Clin. Oncol.* 19 (4): 980–91. PMID 11181660.

[81] Olivotto IA, Bajdik CD, Ravdin PM; et al. (April 2005). "Population-based validation of the prognostic model ADJUVANT! for early breast cancer." *J. Clin. Oncol.* 23 (12): 2716–25. doi:10.1200/JCO. 2005.06. 178. PMID 15837986.

[82] Mook S, Schmidt MK, Rutgers EJ; et al. (November 2009). "Calibration and discriminatory accuracy of prognosis calculation for breast cancer with the online Adjuvant! program: a hospital-based retrospective cohort study." *Lancet Oncol.* 10 (11): 1070–6. doi:10.1016/S1470-2045(09) 70254-2. PMID 19801202.

[83] Campbell HE, Taylor MA, Harris AL, Gray AM (October 2009). "An investigation into the performance of the Adjuvant! Online prognostic programme in early breast cancer for a cohort of patients in the United Kingdom." *Br. J. Cancer* 101 (7): 1074–84. doi:10.1038/sj.bjc.6605283. PMC 2768087. PMID 19724274.

[84] Wishart GC, Azzato EM, Greenberg DC; et al. (2010). "PREDICT: a new UK prognostic model that predicts survival following surgery for invasive breast cancer." *Breast Cancer Res.* 12 (1): R1. doi:10.1186/ bcr2464. PMC 2880419. PMID 20053270.

[85] Dawson SJ, Makretsov N, Blows FM; et al. (August 2010). "BCL2 in breast cancer: a favourable prognostic marker across molecular subtypes and independent of adjuvant therapy received." Br. J. Cancer 103 (5): 668–75. doi:10.1038/sj.bjc.6605736. PMC 2938244. PMID 20664598.

[86] Choosing Treatment for Patients With Ductal Carcinoma In Situ: Fine Tuning the University of Southern California/Van Nuys Prognostic Index Melvin J. Silverstein and Michael D. Lagios *J Natl Cancer Inst Monogr* (2010)2010 (41): 193-196. doi:10.1093/jncimonographs/lgq040.

Chapter 3

Etiopathogenesis of Breast Cancer

Risk Factors in Causation of Breast Cancer

The most important risk factor is gender; only 1% of breast cancer cases occur in men. Common risk factors for women identified by epidemiologic studies have been combined into the Breast Cancer Risk Assessment Tool (BCRAT), which now includes information from the Contraceptive and Reproductive Experiences study [1, 2], which provides more accurate information for African American women. The model can be used to calculate the absolute risk of an individual woman developing invasive cancer within the next 5 years or over a lifetime. The BCRAT incorporates the following risk factors.

Age

The incidence rises throughout a woman's lifetime, peaking at the age of 75–80 years and then declining slightly thereafter. The average age at diagnosis is 61 for white women, 56 for Hispanic women, and 46 for African American women. Only 20% of non-Hispanic white women are diagnosed under the age of 50, compared with 35% of African American women and

31% of Hispanic women. Breast cancer is very rare in all groups before the age of 25.

Although carcinoma is uncommon in young women, almost half of these are either ER negative or human epidermal growth factor receptor 2 (HER2/neu) positive, whereas these cancers make up less than a third of cancers in women over the age of 40.

Age at Menarche

Women who reach menarche when younger than 11 years of age have a 20% increased risk compared with women who are more than 14 years of age at menarche. Late menopause also increases risk.

Age at First Live Birth

Women who experience a first full-term pregnancy at ages younger than 20 years have half the risk of nulliparous women or women over the age of 35 at their first birth. It is hypothesized that pregnancy results in terminal differentiation of milk-producing luminal cells, removing them from the potential pool of cancer precursors [3]. It is also possible that the changes in stroma that allow the growth and expansion of lobules during pregnancy facilitate the transition from in situ to invasive carcinoma. These pregnancy-related changes may help explain the transient increase in cancer risk that follows a pregnancy, an effect that is most pronounced in older women [4].

First-Degree Relatives with Breast Cancer

The risk of breast cancer increases with the number of affected first-degree relatives (mother, sister, or daughter), especially if the cancer occurred at a young age. However, most women do not have a family history. Only 13% of women with breast cancer have one affected first-degree relative, and only 1% has two or more. In turn, over 87% of women with a family history will not develop breast cancer. Most family risk is probably due to the interaction of low-risk susceptibility genes and nongenetic factors. The BCRAT is not designed to calculate the risk for women with a mutation in a high-risk breast cancer gene, such as *BRCA1* or *BRCA2*.

Atypical Hyperplasia

A history of prior breast biopsies, especially if revealing atypical hyperplasia, increases the risk of invasive carcinoma. There is a smaller increase in risk associated with proliferative breast changes without atypia.

Race/Ethnicity

Non-Hispanic white women have the highest rates of breast cancer [5]. However, women of African or Hispanic ancestry present at a more advanced stage and have an increased mortality rate. Social factors such as decreased access to health care and lower use of mammography may well contribute to these disparities, but biologic differences also play an important role [6]. African American and Hispanic women tend to develop cancers at a younger age, prior to menopause, that are more likely to be poorly differentiated and ER negative. Mutations in *p53* are more common in African.

Estrogen Exposure

Postmenopausal hormone replacement therapy increases the risk of breast cancer 1.2- to 1.7-fold, and adding progesterone increases the risk further. Most excess cancers are ER-positive carcinomas [7]. Oral contraceptives have not been shown convincingly to affect breast cancer risk but do decrease the risk of endometrial and ovarian carcinomas. Reducing endogenous estrogens by oophorectomy decreases the risk of developing breast cancer by up to 75%. Drugs that block estrogenic effects (e.g., tamoxifen) or block the formation of estrogen (e.g., aromatase inhibitors) also decrease the risk of ER-positive breast cancer.

Breast Density

High breast radiodensity is a strong risk factor for developing cancer. High density is correlated with young age and hormone exposure, and clusters in families. High breast density may be related to less complete involution of lobules at the end of each menstrual cycle, which in turn may increase the number of cells that are potentially susceptible to neoplastic transformation.

Dense breasts also make detection of cancer more difficult by mammography. Other modalities, such as MRI, may be helpful in such women.

Radiation Exposure

Radiation to the chest, whether due to cancer therapy, atomic bomb exposure, or nuclear accidents, results in a higher rate of breast cancer. The risk is greatest with exposure at young ages and with high radiation doses. For example, women in their teens and early twenty are who received radiation to the chest for Hodgkin lymphomas have a 20% to 30% risk of developing breast cancer over 10 to 30 years. Recognition of this iatrogenic complication has led to a much more judicious use of radiation therapy in adolescents and young women undergoing cancer treatment. The risks of radiation exposure are substantially lower in women over the age of 25. Current mammographic screening uses low doses of radiation and is unlikely to have an effect on the risk of breast cancer.

Carcinoma of the Contralateral Breast or Endometrium

Approximately 1% of women with breast cancer develop a second contralateral breast carcinoma per year. The risk is higher for women with germline mutations in high-risk breast cancer genes such as *BRCA1* and *BRCA2*, who frequently develop multiple cancers. Breast and endometrial carcinomas have several risk factors in common, the most important of which is exposure to prolonged estrogenic stimulation.

Geographic Influence

Breast cancer incidence rates in the United States and Europe are four to seven times higher than those in other countries. Unfortunately, the rates are rising worldwide, and by 2020 it is estimated that 70% of cases will be in developing countries.

The risk of breast cancer increases in immigrants to the United States with each generation. The factors responsible for this increase are of considerable interest because they are likely to include modifiable risk factors.

Reproductive history (number and timing of pregnancies), breastfeeding, diet, obesity, physical activity, and environmental factors all probably play a role.

Diet

Large studies have failed to find strong correlations between breast cancer risk and dietary intake of any specific type of food. Coffee addicts will be pleased to know that caffeine consumption may decrease the risk of breast cancer. On the other hand, moderate or heavy alcohol consumption increases risk. Higher estrogen levels and lower folate levels may underlie this association.

Obesity

There is decreased risk in obese women younger than 40 years as a result of the association with anovulatory cycles and lower progesterone levels late in the cycle. In contrast, the risk is increased for postmenopausal obese women, which is attributed to the synthesis of estrogens in fat depots.

Exercise

There is a probable small protective effect for women who are physically active. The decrease in risk is greatest for premenopausal women, women who are not obese, and women who have had full-term pregnancies.

Breastfeeding

The longer women breastfeed, the greater the reduction in risk. Lactation suppresses ovulation and may trigger terminal differentiation of luminal cells [3]. The lower incidence of breast cancer in developing countries largely can be explained by the more frequent and longer nursing of infants [8].

Environmental Toxins

There is concern that environmental contaminants, such as organochlorine pesticides, have estrogenic effects on humans. Possible links to breast cancer risk are being investigated intensively, but definitive associations have yet to be made.

Tobacco

Cigarette smoking has not been clearly associated with breast cancer but is associated with the development of periductal mastitis (subareolar abscess).

Prevention

Life-Style

Women may reduce their risk of breast cancer by maintaining a healthy weight, drinking less alcohol, being physically active and breastfeeding their children [9]. These modifications might prevent 38% of breast cancers in the US, 42% in the UK, 28% in Brazil and 20% in China [9]. The benefits with moderate exercise such as brisk walking are seen at all age groups including postmenopausal women [9, 10].

Marine omega-3 polyunsaturated fatty acids appear to reduce the risk [11]. Strategies that encourage regular physical activity and reduce obesity could also have other benefits, such as reduced risks of cardiovascular disease and diabetes [13].

High consumption of soy-based foods may reduce risk [12].

Pre-Emptive Surgery

Removal of both breasts before any cancer has been diagnosed or any suspicious lump or other lesion has appeared (a procedure known as prophylactic bilateral mastectomy) may be considered in people with BRCA1 and BRCA2 mutations, which are associated with a substantially heightened risk for an eventual diagnosis of breast cancer [14, 15]. Evidence is not strong enough to support this procedure in anyone but those at the highest risk [16]. BRCA testing is recommended in those with a high family risk after genetic counseling. It is not recommended routinely [17]. This is because there are many forms of changes in *BRCA* genes, ranging from harmless polymorphisms to obviously dangerous frameshift mutations. The effect of most of identifiable changes in the genes is uncertain. Testing in an average-risk person is particularly likely to return one of these indeterminate, useless results. It is unclear if removing the second breast in those who have breast cancer in one is beneficial [16].

Medications

The selective estrogen receptor modulators (such as tamoxifen) reduce the risk of breast cancer but increase the risk of thromboembolism and endometrial cancer [18]. There is no overall change in the risk of death [18, 19]. They are thus not recommended for the prevention of breast cancer in women at average risk but may be offered for those at high risk [20]. The benefit of breast cancer reduction continues for at least five years after stopping a course of treatment with these medications [21].

Etiology and Pathogenesis

The major risk factors for the development of breast cancer are hormonal and genetic. Breast carcinomas can therefore be divided into sporadic cases, probably related to hormonal exposure, and hereditary cases, associated with germline mutations. Hereditary carcinoma has received intense scrutiny in the hopes that the specific genetic mutations can be identified and that these alterations will illuminate the causes of nonfamilial breast cancers as well. Recent studies have borne out these hopes. We begin our discussion with hereditary breast cancer and follow with sporadic breast cancer.

Table 1. Most Common "Single Gene" Mutations Associated with Hereditary Susceptibility to Breast Cancer

GENE (location) Syndrome (Incidence)[*]	% of "Single Gene" Hereditary Cancers[†]	Breast Cancer Risk by Age 70[‡]	Changes in Sporadic Breast Cancer	Other Associated Cancers	Functions	Comments
BRCA1 (17q21) Familial breast and ovarian cancer (1 in 860)	52% (~2% of all breast cancers)	40% to 90%	Mutations rare; inactivated in 50% of some subtypes (e.g., medullary and metaplastic) by methylation	Ovarian, male breast cancer (but lower than BRCA2), prostate, pancreas, fallopian tube	Tumor suppressor, transcriptional regulation, repair of double-stranded DNA breaks	Breast carcinomas are commonly poorly differentiated and triple negative (basal-like), and have *P53* mutations.
BRCA2 (13q12-13) Familial breast and ovarian cancer (1 in 740)	32% (~1% of all breast cancers)	30% to 90%	Mutations and loss of expression rare	Ovarian, male breast cancer, prostate, pancreas, stomach, melanoma, gallbladder, bile duct, pharynx	Tumor suppressor, transcriptional regulation, repair of double-stranded DNA breaks	Biallelic germline mutations cause a rare form of Fanconi anemia.

GENE (location) Syndrome (Incidence)[*]	% of "Single Gene" Hereditary Cancers[†]	Breast Cancer Risk by Age 70[‡]	Changes in Sporadic Breast Cancer	Other Associated Cancers	Functions	Comments
p53 (17p13.1) Li-Fraumeni (1 in 5,000)	3% (<1% of all breast cancers)	>90%	Mutations in 20%, LOH in 30% to 42%; most frequent in triple negative cancers	Sarcoma, leukemia, brain tumors, adrenocortical carcinoma, others	Tumor suppressor with critical roles in cell cycle control, DNA replication, DNA repair, and apoptosis	*p53* is the most commonly mutated gene in sporadic breast cancers
CHEK2 (22q12.1) Li-Fraumeni variant (1 in 100)	5% (~1% of all breast cancers)	10% to 20%	Mutations rare (<5%); loss of protein expression in at least one third by unknown mechanism(s)	Prostate, thyroid, kidney, colon	Cell cycle checkpoint kinase, recognition and repair of DNA damage, activates BRCA1 and p53 by phosphorylation	May increase risk for breast cancer after radiation exposure

* Frequency of heterozygotes in the U.S. population; the incidence of gene mutations is higher in some ethnic populations (e.g., BRCA1 and BRCA2 mutations occur at high frequencies in Askenazi Jews).

† Defined as familial breast cancers showing a pattern of inheritance consistent with a major effect of a single gene.

‡ Risk varies with specific mutations and is likely modified by other genes.

Hereditary Breast Cancer

The inheritance of a susceptibility gene or genes is the primary cause of approximately 12% of breast cancers [22, 23]. The probability of a hereditary etiology increases with multiple affected first-degree relatives, when individuals are affected before menopause and/or have multiple cancers, or there are family members with other specific cancers.

In some families the increased risk is the result of a single mutation in a highly penetrant breast cancer gene (Table 1). Mutations in *BRCA1* and *BRCA2* account for the majority of cancers attributable to single mutations and about 3% of all breast cancers. Penetrance (the percentage of carriers who develop breast cancer) varies from 30% to 90% depending on the specific mutation present. Mutations in *BRCA1* also markedly increase the risk of developing ovarian carcinoma, which occurs in as many as 20% to 40% of carriers. *BRCA2* confers a smaller risk for ovarian carcinoma (10% to 20%) but is associated more frequently with male breast cancer. *BRCA1* and *BRCA2* carriers are also at higher risk for other epithelial cancers, such as prostatic and pancreatic carcinomas.

BRCA1 and *BRCA2* are both large genes over 80 kilobases in size. Hundreds of different mutations distributed throughout the coding regions have been reported for each. The frequency of mutations that increase breast cancer risk is only 0.1% to 0.2% in the general population, and inconsequential polymorphisms are common. As a result, genetic testing is difficult and generally restricted to individuals with a strong family history or those belonging to certain ethnic groups. For example, 2% to 3% of people of Ashkenazi Jewish descent carry one of three specific mutations, two in *BRCA1* and one in *BRCA2*. Identification of carriers is important, since increased surveillance, prophylactic mastectomy, and oophorectomy can reduce cancer-related morbidity and mortality.

BRCA1-associated breast cancers are commonly poorly differentiated, have "medullary features" (a syncytial growth pattern with pushing margins and a lymphocytic response), and do not express hormone receptors or overexpress HER2/neu (the so-called "triple negative" phenotype). Their gene profiling signature is very similar to basal-like breast cancers, a distinct molecular subtype that is discussed later. *BRCA1* cancers are also frequently associated with loss of the inactive X chromosome and reduplication of the active X, resulting in the absence of the Barr body [25]. *BRCA2*-associated breast carcinomas also tend to be relatively poorly differentiated, but are more often ER positive than *BRCA1* cancers.

Other known susceptibility genes are much less commonly implicated; together, this group accounts for fewer than 10% of hereditary breast carcinomas. Li-Fraumeni syndrome (due to germline mutations in *p53*) and Li-Fraumeni variant syndrome (due to germline mutations in *CHEK2*) together account for about 8% of breast cancers caused by single genes. Three other tumor suppressor genes, ***PTEN*** (Cowden syndrome), ***LKBI/STK11*** (Peutz-Jeghers syndrome), and ***ATM*** (ataxia telangiectasia), are mutated in less than 1% of all breast cancers.

Sporadic Breast Cancer

The major risk factors for sporadic breast cancer are related to hormone exposure: gender, age at menarche and menopause, reproductive history, breastfeeding, and exogenous estrogens. The majority of sporadic cancers occurs in postmenopausal women and is ER positive.

Hormonal exposure increases the number of potential target cells by stimulating breast growth during puberty, menstrual cycles, and pregnancy. Exposure also drives cycles of proliferation that place cells at risk for DNA damage. Once premalignant or malignant cells are present, hormones can stimulate their growth, as well as the growth of normal epithelial and stromal cells that may aid and abet tumor development.

Estrogen may also play a more direct role in carcinogenesis. **Metabolites of estrogen can cause mutations or generate DNA-damaging free radicals in cell** and animal model systems [25]. It also has been proposed that variants of genes involved in estrogen synthesis and metabolism could increase the risk of breast cancer. Such variants would be analogous to cytochrome P-450 alleles that alter the metabolism of tamoxifen in some women [26].

Overview of Carcinogenesis and Tumor Progression

The diverse histologic appearances of carcinomas and putative precursor lesions are the outward manifestations of the complex genetic and epigenetic changes that drive carcinogenesis. One model of carcinogenesis postulates that a normal cell must acquire several new capabilities to become malignant [27, 28]. Each may be achieved by a change in the activity of one of many different genes that regulate common cellular activities.

Populations of cells that harbor some, but not all, of the genetic and epigenetic changes that are required for carcinogenesis give rise to morphologically recognizable breast lesions (discussed earlier) that are associated with an increased risk of progression to cancer. The earliest such alterations are proliferative changes, which may stem from the loss of growth-inhibiting signals, aberrant increases in pro-growth signals, or decreased apoptosis. For example, most early lesions (such as atypical ductal hyperplasia and atypical lobular hyperplasia) show increased expression of hormone receptors and abnormal regulation of proliferation [37, 29]. LOH is rarely detected in typical proliferative change but becomes more frequent in atypical hyperplasias and is almost universally present in carcinoma in situ. Profound DNA instability in the form of aneuploidy, which manifests morphologically by nuclear enlargement, irregularity, and hyperchromasia, is observed only in high-grade DCIS and some invasive carcinomas. At some point during tumor progression the malignant clone also becomes immortalized and acquires the ability to drive neo-angiogenesis. The morphologic and biologic features of carcinomas are usually established at the in situ stage, since in the majority of cases the in situ lesion closely resembles the accompanying invasive carcinoma.

The cell of origin of breast cancers is of interest, since this has important implications for etiology and treatment. The "cancer stem cell hypothesis" proposes that malignant changes occur in a stem cell population that has unique properties distinguishing them from more differentiated cells [30, 31]. Although the majority of tumor cells would consist of non–stem cell progeny, only the malignant stem cells would contribute to tumor progression or recurrence. Effective treatment would need to target only this population, which to date has been difficult to define.

The most likely cell type of origin for the majority of carcinomas is the ER-expressing luminal cell, since the majority of cancers are ER-positive and precursor lesions, such as atypical hyperplasias, are most similar to this type of cell. ER-negative carcinomas may arise from ER-negative myoepithelial cells [32, 33]. This would explain why many proteins found in myoepithelial cells are shared by the "triple-negative" or basal-like cancers. An alternative possibility is an origin from an ER-positive precursor that loses ER expression [37, 34]. The precursor lesion for ER-negative tumors is unknown.

The final step of carcinogenesis, the transition of carcinoma in situ to invasive carcinoma, is the most important and unfortunately the least understood. Genetic markers specific for invasive carcinomas have been difficult to identify. It is important to remember that the structure and function of the normal breast depend on a complex interplay between luminal cells, myoepithelial cells, and stromal cells. The same molecular events that allow for the normal formation of new ductal branch points and lobules during puberty and pregnancy—abrogation of the basement membrane, increased proliferation, escape from growth inhibition, angiogenesis, and invasion of stroma—may be recapitulated during carcinogenesis [38]. Remodeling of the breast, which involves inflammatory and "wound healing–like" tissue reactions, could explain the transient increase in breast cancers during and shortly after pregnancy, since such changes could facilitate the transition of carcinoma in situ to invasive cancer [4, 35, 36].

As can be summarized from this discussion, there are many paths that can lead to the development of breast cancer. Breast cancer is not one disease, but many, each with its own clinical characteristics and optimal prevention and treatment strategies.

References

[1] Gail MH, et al: Projecting individualized probabilities of developing breast cancer for white females who are being examined annually. *J Natl Cancer Inst* 1989; 81:1879.

[2] Gail MH, et al: Projecting individualized absolute invasive breast cancer risk in African American women. *J Natl Cancer Inst* 2007; 99:1782.

[3] Russo J, et al: Full-term pregnancy induces a specific genomic signature in the human breast. *Cancer Epidemiol Biomarkers Prev* 2008; 17:51.

[4] Schedin P: Pregnancy-associated breast cancer and metastasis. *Nat Rev Cancer* 2006; 4:281.

[5] Morris CR, et al: The risk of developing breast cancer within the next 5, 10, or 20 years of a woman's life. *Am J Prev Med* 2001; 20:213.

[6] Hayanga AJ, Newman LA: Investigating the phenotypes and genotypes of breast cancer in women with African ancestry: the need for more genetic epidemiology. *Surg Clin North Am* 2007; 87:551.

[7] Rossouw JE, et al: Risks and benefits of estrogen plus progestin in healthy postmenopausal women: principal results from the Women's Health Initiative randomized controlled trial. *JAMA* 2002; 288:321.

[8] Beral VCollaborative Group on Hormonal Factors in Breast Cancer: Breast cancer and breastfeeding: collaborative reanalysis of individual data from 47 epidemiological studies in 30 countries, including 50,302

women with breast cancer and 96,973 women without the disease. *Lancet* 2002; 360:187.

[9] American Institute for Cancer Research/World Cancer Research Fund, Food, Nutrition, Physical Activity and the Prevention of Cancer: a Global Perspective.

[10] Eliassen AH, Hankinson SE, Rosner B, Holmes MD, Willett WC (October 2010). "Physical activity and risk of breast cancer among postmenopausal women." *Arch. Intern. Med.* 170 (19): 1758–64. doi:10.1001/archinternmed.2010.363. PMC 3142573. PMID 20975025.

[11] Zheng JS, Hu XJ, Zhao YM, Yang J, Li D (2013). "Intake of fish and marine n-3 polyunsaturated fatty acids and risk of breast cancer: meta-analysis of data from 21 independent prospective cohort studies." *BMJ* 346: f3706. doi:10.1136/bmj.f3706. PMID 23814120.

[12] Wu, AH; Yu, MC; Tseng, CC; Pike, MC (15 January 2008). "Epidemiology of soy exposures and breast cancer risk." *British journal of cancer* 98 (1): 9–14. doi:10.1038/sj.bjc.6604145. PMID 18182974.

[13] "SEER Stat Fact Sheets: Breast Cancer." NCI. Retrieved 18 June 2014.

[14] Hartmann LC, Schaid DJ, Woods JE, Crotty TP, Myers JL, Arnold PG, Petty PM, Sellers TA, Johnson JL, McDonnell SK, Frost MH, Jenkins RB (1999). "Efficacy of bilateral prophylactic mastectomy in women with a family history of breast cancer." *N Engl J Med* 340 (2): 77–84. doi:10.1056/NEJM199901143400201. PMID 9887158.

[15] Meijers-Heijboer H, van Geel B, van Putten WL, Henzen-Logmans SC, Seynaeve C, Menke-Pluymers MB, Bartels CC, Verhoog LC, van den Ouweland AM, Niermeijer MF, Brekelmans CT, Klijn JG (2001). "Breast cancer after prophylactic bilateral mastectomy in women with BRCA1 and BRCA2 mutations." *N Engl J Med* 345 (3): 159–164. doi:10.1056/NEJM200107193450301. PMID 11463009.

[16] Lostumbo, L; Carbine, NE; Wallace, J (10 November 2010). "Prophylactic mastectomy for the prevention of breast cancer." The Cochrane database of systematic reviews (11): CD002748. doi:10.1002/14651858.CD002748.pub3. PMID 21069671.

[17] "Risk Assessment, Genetic Counseling, and Genetic Testing for BRCA-Related Cancer in Women: U.S. Preventive Services Task Force Recommendation Statement." *Annals of Internal Medicine* 160: 271–281. 24 December 2013. doi:10.7326/M13-2747.

[18] Nelson HD, Smith ME, Griffin JC, Fu R (16 April 2013). "Use of medications to reduce risk for primary breast cancer: a systematic review for the U.S. Preventive Services Task Force." *Annals of Internal*

Medicine 158 (8): 604–14. doi:10.7326/0003-4819-158-8-201304160-00005. PMID 23588749.

[19] Cuzick J, Sestak I, Bonanni B, Costantino JP, Cummings S, DeCensi A, Dowsett M, Forbes JF, Ford L, LaCroix AZ, Mershon J, Mitlak BH, Powles T, Veronesi U, Vogel V, Wickerham DL (25 May 2013). "Selective oestrogen receptor modulators in prevention of breast cancer: an updated meta-analysis of individual participant data." *Lancet* 381 (9880): 1827–34. doi:10.1016/S0140-6736(13)60140-3. PMID 2363 9488.

[20] Moyer VA (24 September 2013). "Medications for Risk Reduction of Primary Breast Cancer in Women: U.S. Preventive Services Task Force Recommendation Statement." *Annals of Internal Medicine*. doi:10.7326/0003-4819-159-10-201311190-00718. PMID 24061472.

[21] Cuzick J, Sestak I, Bonanni B, Costantino JP, Cummings S, DeCensi A, Dowsett M, Forbes JF, Ford L, LaCroix AZ, Mershon J, Mitlak BH, Powles T, Veronesi U, Vogel V, Wickerham DL (31 March 2013). "Selective oestrogen receptor modulators in prevention of breast cancer: an updated meta-analysis of individual participant data." *The Lancet* 381 (9880): 1827–34. doi:10.1016/S0140-6736(13)60140-3. PMID 23639488.

[22] Bradbury AR, Olopade OI: Genetic susceptibility to breast cancer. *Rev Endocr Metab Disord* 2007; 8:225.

[23] Garcia-Closas M, et al: Heterogeneity of breast cancer associations with five susceptibility loci by clinical and pathological characteristics. *PLOS Genetics* 2008; 4:e10000054.

[24] Pageau GJ, et al: The disappearing Barr body in breast and ovarian cancers. *Nat Rev Cancer* 2007; 7:628.

[25] Yager JD, Davidson NE: Estrogen carcinogenesis in breast cancer. *N Engl J Med* 2006; 354:270.

[26] Desta Z, Flockhart DA: Germline pharmacogenetics of tamoxifen response: have we learned enough?. *J Clin Oncol* 2007; 25:5147.

[27] Hanahan D, Weinberg RA: The hallmarks of cancer. *Cell* 2000; 100:57.

[28] Hahn WC, Weinberg RA: Rules for making human tumor cells. *N Engl J Med* 2002; 347:1593.

[29] Iqbal M, et al: Subgroups of non-atypical hyperplasia of breast defined by proliferation of oestrogen receptor-positive cells. *J Pathol* 2001; 193:333.

[30] Campbell LL, Polyak K: Breast tumor heterogeneity. Cancer stem cells or clonal evolution?. *Cell Cycle* 2007; 6:2332.

[31] Stingl J, Caldas C: Molecular heterogeneity of breast carcinomas and the cancer stem cell hypothesis. *Nat Rev Cancer* 2007; 10:791.

[32] Murad TM: A proposed histochemical and electron microscopic classification of human breast cancer according to cell of origin. *Cancer* 1971; 27:288.

[33] Shipitisin M, et al: Molecular definition of breast tumor heterogeneity. *Cancer Cell* 2007; 11:259.

[34] Gauthier ML, et al: Abrogated response to cellular stress identifies DCIS associated with subsequent tumor events and defines basal-like breast tumors. *Cancer Cell* 2007; 12:479.

[35] Tlsty T, Coussens LM: Tumor stroma and regulation of cancer development. *Ann Rev Pathol Mech Dis* 2006; 1:119.

[36] Patocs A, et al: Breast-cancer stromal cells with TP53 mutations and nodal metastases. *N Engl J Med* 2007; 357:2543.

[37] Allred DC, et al: Ductal carcinoma in situ and the emergence of diversity during breast cancer evolution. *Clin Cancer Res* 2008; 14:370.

[38] Wiseman BS, Werb Z: Stromal effects on mammary gland development and breast cancer. *Science* 2002; 296:1046.

Chapter 4

In Situ Breast Cancer

Ductal Carcinoma in Situ (DCIS)

Epidemiology

"*DCIS is often detected with mammographies but can rarely be felt.*" With the increasing use of screening mammography, noninvasive cancers are more frequently diagnosed and now constitute 15% to 20% of all breast cancers [33].

Cases of DCIS have increased 5 fold between 1983 and 2003 in the United States due to the introduction of screening mammography [30]. In 2009 about 62,000 cases were diagnosed [30].

Causes

The specific causes of DCIS are still unknown. The risk factors for developing this condition are similar to those for invasive breast cancer [17].

Some women are however more prone than others to developing DCIS. Women considered at higher risks are those who have a family history of breast cancer, those who have had their periods at an early age or who have had a late menopause. Also, women who have never had children or had them late in life are also more likely to get this condition.

Long-term use of estrogen-progestin hormone replacement therapy (HRT) for more than five years after menopause, genetic mutations (BRCA1 or

BRCA2 genes), atypical hyperplasia, as well as radiation exposure or exposure to certain chemicals may also contribute in the development of the condition [18]. Nonetheless, the risk of developing noninvasive cancer increases with age and it is higher in women older than 45 years.

Terminology

Ductal carcinoma in situ (DCIS) is the name given to groups of "cancerous" epithelial cells that have remained in their normal place (in situ in Latin) within the ducts and lobules of the mammary gland (Figures 1 and 2) [10]. Clinically, it is considered a premalignant (i.e., potentially malignant) condition [11]. Each lesion contains cells that have already become biologically malignant (cancerous) but have not yet crossed the basement membrane to invade the surrounding tissue [10, 12]. When multiple lesions (known as "foci" of DCIS) are present in different quadrants of the breast, this is referred to as "multicentric" disease [6].

For statistical purposes, some count DCIS as a "cancer," whereas others do not [9, 13]. When classified as a cancer, it is referred to as a non-invasive or pre-invasive form [10, 14]. The National Cancer Institute describes it as a "noninvasive condition [9].

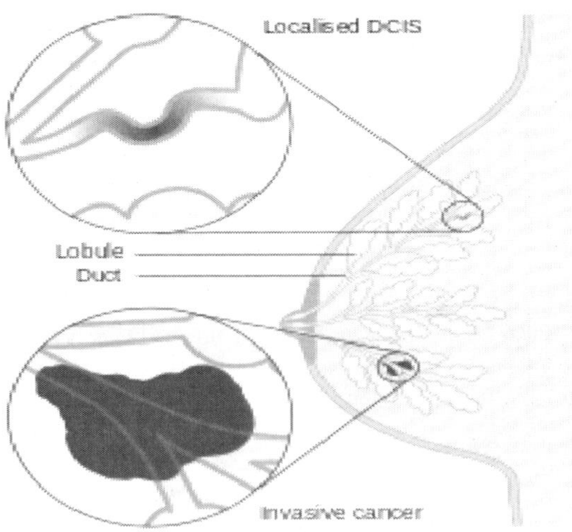

Figure 1. Showing a drawing of ductal carcinoma in situ in the anatomical context of the whole breast.

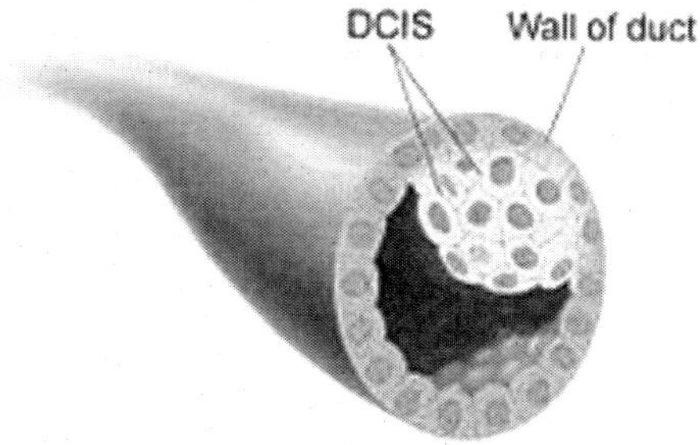

Figure 2. Showing a drawing of a breast duct containing ductal carcinoma in situ.

Signs and Symptoms

Most of the women who develop DCIS do not experience any symptoms. The first signs and symptoms may appear if the cancer advances. Because of the lack of early symptoms, DCIS is most often detected at screening mammography.

In a few cases, DCIS may cause:

- A lump or thickening in or near the breast or under the arm
- A change in the size or shape of the breast
- Nipple discharge or nipple tenderness; the nipple may also be inverted, or pulled back into the breast
- Ridges or pitting of the breast; the skin may look like the skin of an orange
- A change in the way the skin of the breast, areola, or nipple looks or feels [15] such as warmth, swelling, redness or scaliness [16].

Diagnosis

80% of cases in the United States are diagnosed by mammography screening [19].

On FNAC:- high grade DCIS shows large pleomorphic cells with malignant features in sheets, irregular aggregates and singles and low grade DCIS shows mild to moderate epithelial cells mainly cohesive, forming large sheets often with holes or papillary fragments [35].

Following table shows the difference between the epithelial hyperplasia, ADH and low grade DCIS on FNAC study [36].

Epithelial hyperplasia	Atypical hyperplasia	Low grade DCIS
Cell rich smear, large sheets of cohesive epithelial cells, few single cells.	Cell rich smear, large sheets of cohesive epithelial cells, few single cells.	Cell rich smear, large sheets of cohesive epithelial cells, few single cells.
Cells often in streaming pattern, focal crowding and overlapping of nuclei rarely 'holes.'	Focal crowding and overlapping of nuclei, 'holes suggestive of cribriform pattern in some cases.	Focal crowding and overlapping of nuclei, 'holes suggestive of cribriform pattern common, some papillary cell groups.
Nuclear atypia absent or mild.	Mild to moderate nuclear atypia.	Mild to moderate nuclear atypia.
Naked bipolar and myoepithelial nuclei present but may be few, clean background, calcium granules occasionally.	Naked bipolar and myoepithelial nuclei present, debris and calcium granules occasionally present.	Naked bipolar and myoepithelial nuclei absent, necrotic debris and calcium often but not invariably present.

Variants of DCIS include:

1. Comedocarcinoma- It is a grade 3 DCIS grossly tumor present as cluster of thick wall duct with normal breast parenchyma between them. When this duct are compressed plugs of necrotic tumor reminiscent-like comedons extrude from them, hence the name comedocarcinoma. Microscopically duct shows solid growth of large pleomorphic tumor cells with abundant mitotic activity and lacking connective tissue support, necrosis always present. Stroma may show fibrosis with inflammation (Figures 3 and 4).

2. **In situ papillary carcinoma**- Grossly it is well circumscribed mass or may ramify within several ducts to involve an entire breast segment Microscopically tumor shows uniformity in size and shape of epithelial cell (whether round, oval, spindle), presence of one cell type only (i.e, lack of myoepithelial cell), nuclear hyperchromasia & high nucleocytoplasmic ratio, high mitotic activity (Figure 5). It may show lack of apocrine metaplasia, cribriform & trabecular pattern. Scattered large pale eosinophilic (clear/globoid cells) are also seen, which are immunoreactive for GCDFP-15. Variants include intracystic type, solid variant, transitional type and encapsulated apocrine papillary carcinoma.

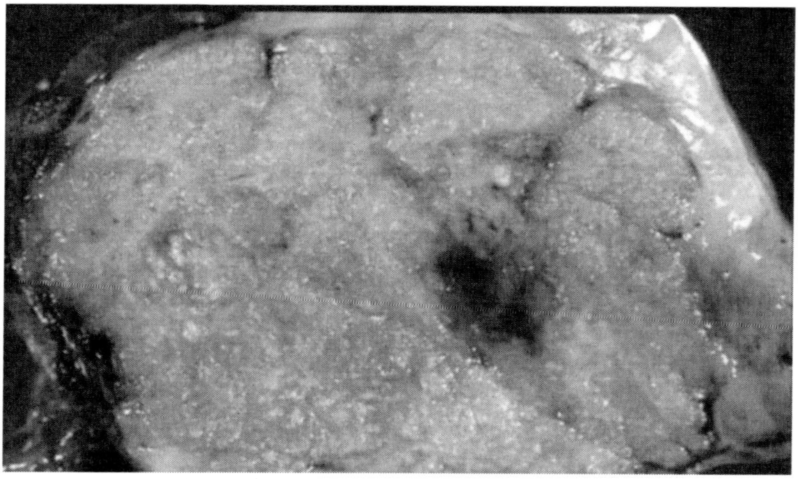

Figure 3. Gross of comedocarcinoma.

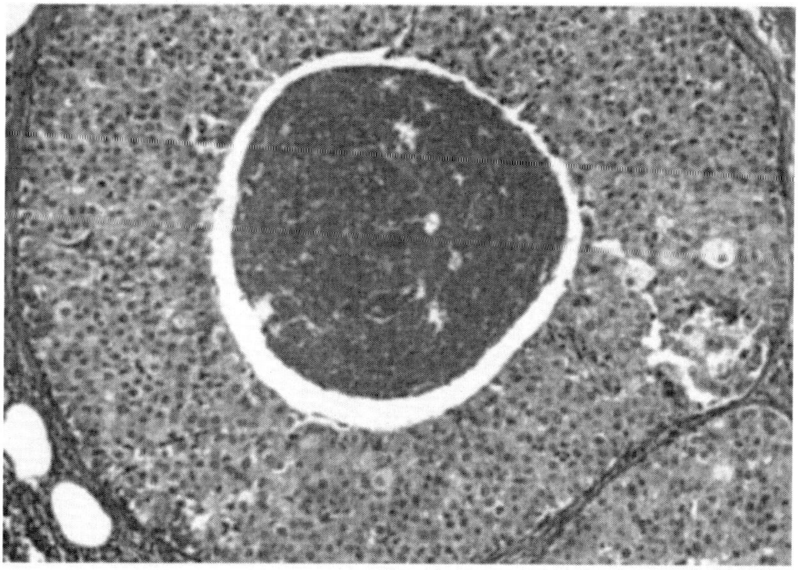

Figure 4. Showing microscopy comedocarcinoma.

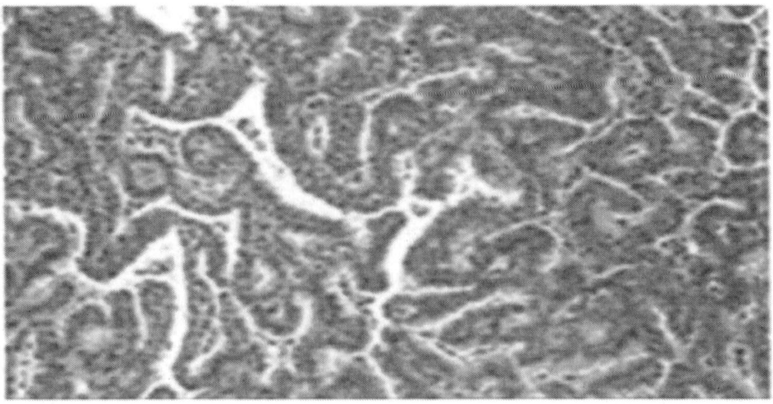

Figure 5. Gross and microscopy showing papillary carcinoma.

3. **Solid variant**:- Glandular lumen filled by proliferation of medium sized cells (Figure 6).

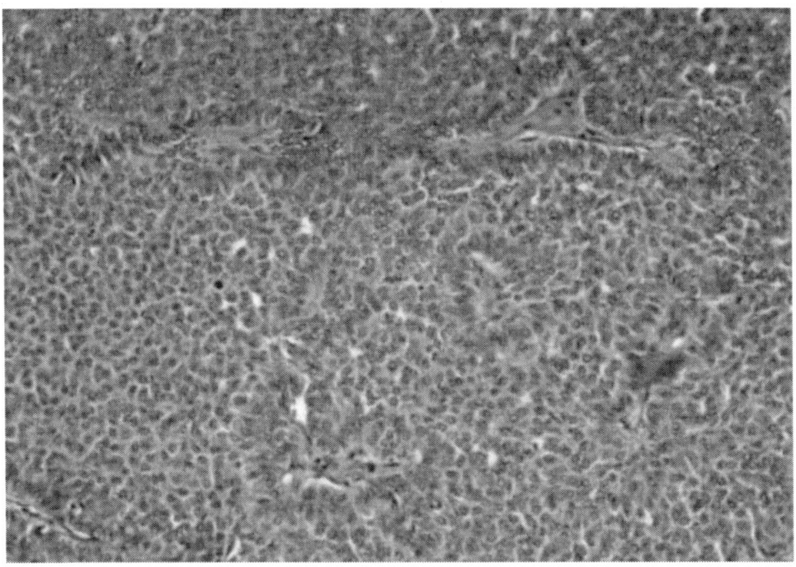

Figure 6. Showing solid sheets of tumor cells.

4. **Cribriform DCIS:-** round regular spaces formed within the glands, more regular these spaces and size shape more the lesion is malignant (Figure 7). It shows trabecular bars and roman bridges. It is differentiated from adenoid cystic carcinoma.

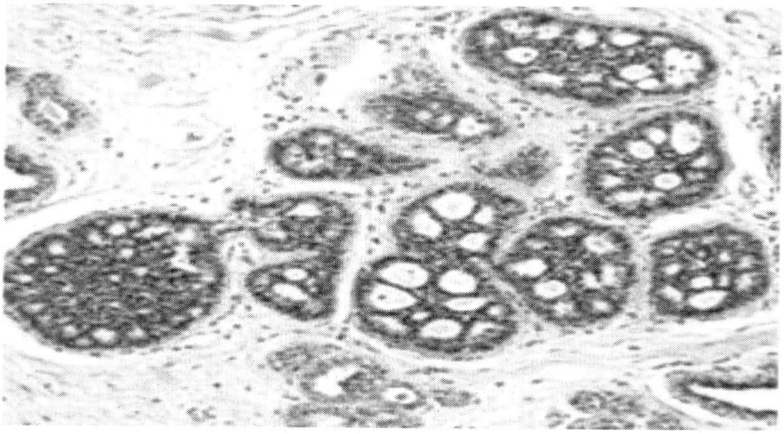

Figure 7. Showing cribriform cellular arrangement.

5. **Micropapillary variety:-** shows elongated epithelial projections projecting into the glandular lumen (Figure 8).

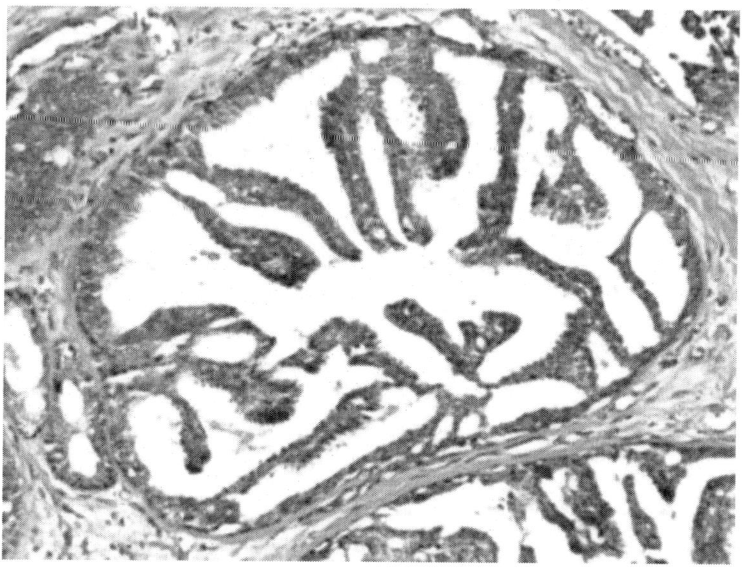

Figure 8. Showing micropapillary pattern in glandular lumen.

6. **Clinging carcinoma:-** shows one to two layer of malignant cell lining a glandular formation with a large empty lumen may show granular intraluminal material with ghost of tumor cells identified (Figure 9).

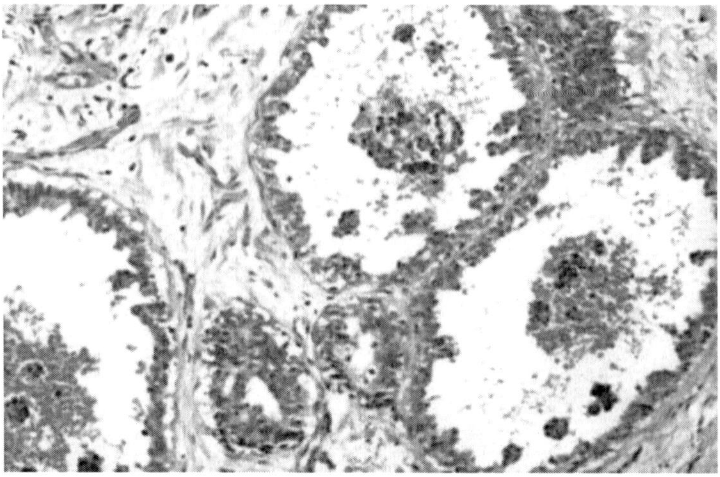

Figure 9. Showing malignant cells lining glandular formation.

7. **Cystic hypersecretory:-** Cystic formation induced by the abundant secretory material present (Figure 10).

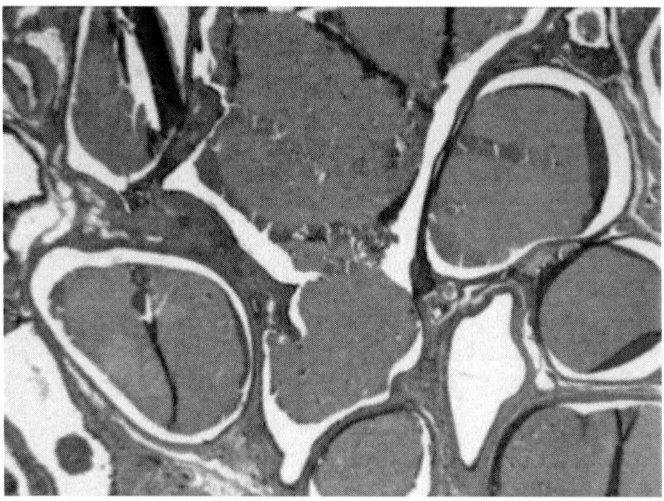

Figure 10. Showing cystic hypersecretory.

Histopathological Features diagnostic important to diagnose DCIS:-

- Appearance of luminal content
- Nuclear debris

- Ghost of dead cell outline
- Granular and fragmented products
- Inspissated densely stained material.

IHC positive for E-cadherin and scantiness or absence of HMW keratin. High grade DCIS also shows P- cadherin (Figure 11) [34].

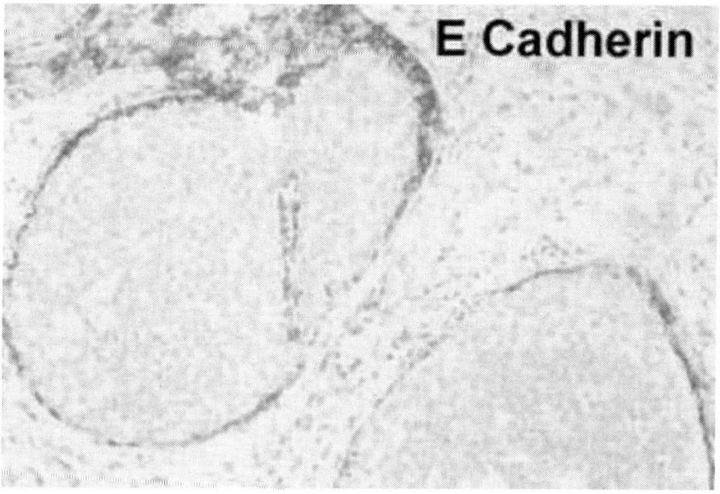

Figure 11. IHC showing E cadherin positivity.

Treatment

Surgical removal, with or without additional radiation therapy or tamoxifen, is the recommended treatment for DCIS [20]. Surgery may be either a breast-conserving lumpectomy or a mastectomy (complete or partial removal of the affected breast) [21]. If a lumpectomy is used it is often combined with radiation therapy [9]. Tamoxifen may be used as hormonal therapy if the cells show estrogen receptor positivity [9]. Chemotherapy is not needed for DCIS since the disease is noninvasive [22].

While surgery reduces the risk of subsequent cancer, many people never develop cancer even without treatment and there are associated side effects [21]. There is no evidence comparing surgery with watchful waiting and some feel watchful waiting may be a reasonable option in certain cases [21].

Radiation Therapy

Use of radiation therapy after lumpectomy provides equivalent survival rates to mastectomy, although here is a slightly higher risk of recurrent disease in the same breast in the form of further DCIS or invasive breast cancer. Systematic reviews (including a Cochrane review) indicate that the addition of radiation therapy to lumpectomy reduces recurrence of DCIS or later onset of invasive breast cancer in comparison with breast-conserving surgery alone, without affecting mortality [23, 24]. The Cochrane review did not find any evidence that the radiation therapy had any long-term toxic effects [23]. While the authors caution that longer follow-up will be required before a definitive conclusion can be reached regarding long-term toxicity, they point out that ongoing technical improvements should further restrict radiation exposure in healthy tissues [23]. They do recommend that comprehensive information on potential side effects is given to women who receive this treatment [23]. The addition of radiation therapy to lumpectomy appears to reduce the risk of local recurrence to approximately 12%, of which approximately half will be DCIS and half will be invasive breast cancer; the risk of recurrence is 1% for women undergoing mastectomy [25].

Mastectomy

There is no evidence that mastectomy decreases the risk of death over a lumpectomy [26]. Mastectomy; however, may decrease the rate of the DCIS or invasive cancer occurring in the same location [26].

Mastectomies remain a common recommendation in those with persistent microscopic involvement of margins after local excision or with a diagnosis of DCIS and evidence of suspicious, diffuse microcalcifications [27]. Some institutions that have encountered high rates of recurrent invasive cancers after mastectomy for DCIS have endorsed routine sentinel node biopsy (SNB) [28]. Others reserve SNB for only certain people. Most agree that SNB should be considered with tissue diagnosis of high risk DCIS (grade III with palpable mass or larger size on imaging) as well as in people undergoing mastectomy after a core or excisional biopsy diagnosis of DCIS [29].

Prognosis

Because DCIS is normally found early and it is treated or managed, it is difficult to say what occurs if left untreated. About 2% of women who are diagnosed with this condition and treated died within 10 years [30]. Biomarkers can identify which women who were initially diagnosed with DCIS are at high or low risk of subsequent invasive cancer [31, 32].

References

[1] Sinn, HP; Kreipe, H (May 2013). "A Brief Overview of the WHO Classification of Breast Tumors, 4th Edition, Focusing on Issues and Updates from the 3rd Edition." Breast care (Basel, Switzerland) 8 (2): 149–154. doi:10.1159/000350774. PMID 24415964.

[2] Seltzer, William H. Hindle, editor; with a foreword by Vicki (1999). Breast care: a clinical guidebook for women's primary health care providers. New York: Springer. p. 129. ISBN 9780387983486.

[3] Staging, Breastcancer.org.

[4] Welch HG, Woloshin S, Schwartz LM (February 2008). "The sea of uncertainty surrounding ductal carcinoma in situ--the price of screening mammography." *J. Natl. Cancer Inst.* 100 (4): 228–9. doi:10.1093/jnci/djn013. PMID 18270336.

[5] Liberman, Laura (2005). Breast MRI. [New York]: Springer Science+Business Media, Inc. p. 164. ISBN 9780387219974.

[6] Virnig BA, Shamliyan T, Tuttle TM, Kane RL, Wilt TJ (September 2009). "Diagnosis and management of ductal carcinoma in situ (DCIS)." Evidence Report/Technology Assessment. AHRQ Publication No.09-E018. (185): 1–549. PMID 20629475.

[7] Rubin's Pathology: clinicopathologic foundations of medicine (5. ed.). Philadelphia [u.a.]: Wolters Kluwer/Lippincott Williams & Wilkins. 2008. p. 848. ISBN 9780781795166. |first1= missing |last1= in Authors list (help)

[8] "Breast Cancer Treatment (PDQ®)." NCI. 2014-04-11. Retrieved 19 June 2014.

[9] "Breast Cancer Treatment (PDQ®)." NCI. Retrieved 19 June 2014.

[10] Allred DC (2010). "Ductal carcinoma in situ: terminology, classification, and natural history." *Journal of the National Cancer*

Institute. Monographs 2010 (41): 134–8. doi:10.1093/jncimonographs/lgq035. PMID 20956817.

[11] Padwal, David Hui (2011). Alexander Leung and Raj Padwal, ed. Approach to internal medicine a resource book for clinical practice (3rd ed.). New York: *Springer*. p. 198. ISBN 9781441965059.

[12] Tjandra, Joe J.; Collins, John P. (2006). "Breast surgery." In Tjandra; et al. Textbook of surgery (3rd ed.). *Malden, Mass.:* Blackwell Pub. p. 282. ISBN 9780470757796.

[13] Chang, Alfred (2007). Oncology: An Evidence-Based Approach. *Springer*. p. 162. ISBN 9780387310565.

[14] J.@Saclarides, ed. by Jonathan A.@Myers, Keith W.@Millikan, Theodore (2008). Common surgical diseases an algorithmic approach to problem solving. (2nd rev. ed.). New York: *Springer*. ISBN 9780387752464.

[15] "Breast Cancer." Retrieved 2010-06-28.

[16] "Signs and Symptoms." Retrieved 2010-06-28.

[17] "After the mammogram." Retrieved 2010-06-28.

[18] "Intraductal Carcinoma of the Breast." Retrieved 2010-06-28.

[19] "Ductal Carcinoma In Situ." cancer.gov. January 9, 2015. Retrieved 5 March 2015.

[20] "Ductal Carcinoma In Situ: Treatment Options for Patients With DCIS." National Cancer Institute at NIH. National Institutes of Health. 2014-07-11.

[21] "Treatment of ductal carcinoma in situ: an uncertain harm-benefit balance." *Prescrire Int* 144 (22): 298–303. Dec 2013. PMID 24600734.

[22] Ductal Carcinoma in Situ (DCIS), Johns Hopkins Medicine.

[23] Goodwin A, Parker S, Ghersi D, Wilcken N (2013). "Post-operative radiotherapy for ductal carcinoma in situ of the breast." The Cochrane Database of Systematic Reviews 11: CD000563. doi:10.1002/14651858.CD000563.pub7. PMID 24259251.

[24] Virnig, BA; Tuttle, TM; Shamliyan, T; Kane, RL (2010). "Ductal carcinoma in situ of the breast: a systematic review of incidence, treatment, and outcomes." *Journal of the National Cancer Institute* 102 (3): 170–8. doi:10.1093/jnci/djp482. PMID 20071685.

[25] "NIH DCIS Consensus Conference Statement." National Institutes of Health. September 2009.

[26] Virnig, BA; Shamliyan, T; Tuttle, TM; Kane, RL; Wilt, TJ (September 2009). "Diagnosis and management of ductal carcinoma in situ (DCIS)." Evidence report/technology assessment (185): 4. PMID 20629475. They

found women undergoing mastectomy were less likely than women undergoing lumpectomy plus radiation to experience local DCIS or invasive recurrence. Women undergoing BCS alone were also more likely to experience a local recurrence than women treated with mastectomy. We found no study showing a mortality reduction associated with mastectomy over breast conserving surgery with or without radiation.

[27] "Intraductal carcinoma." Retrieved 2010-06-28.

[28] Tan JC, McCready DR, Easson AM, Leong WL (February 2007). "Role of sentinel lymph node biopsy in ductal carcinoma-in-situ treated by mastectomy." *Annals of Surgical Oncology* 14 (2): 638–45. doi:10.1245/s10434-006-9211-9. PMID 17103256.

[29] van Deurzen CH, Hobbelink MG, van Hillegersberg R, van Diest PJ (April 2007). "Is there an indication for sentinel node biopsy in patients with ductal carcinoma in situ of the breast? A review." *European Journal of Cancer* 43 (6): 993–1001. doi:10.1016/j.ejca.2007.01.010. PMID 17300928.

[30] Kerlikowske, K (2010). "Epidemiology of ductal carcinoma in situ." *Journal of the National Cancer Institute*. Monographs 2010 (41): 139–41. doi:10.1093/jncimonographs/lgq027. PMID 20956818.

[31] Kerlikowske, K.; Molinaro, A. M.; Gauthier, M. L.; Berman, H. K.; Waldman, F.; Bennington, J.; Sanchez, H.; Jimenez, C.; Stewart, K.; et al. (2010). "Biomarker Expression and Risk of Subsequent Tumors After Initial Ductal Carcinoma in Situ Diagnosis." *JNCI Journal of the National Cancer Institute* 102 (9): 627–637. doi:10.1093/jnci/djq101. PMC 2864293. PMID 20427430.

[32] Witkiewicz AK, Dasgupta A, Nguyen KH, et al. (June 2009). "Stromal caveolin-1 levels predict early DCIS progression to invasive breast cancer." *Cancer Biology & Therapy* 8 (11): 1071–1079. doi:10.4161/cbt.8.11.8874. PMID 19502809.

[33] "Intraductal carcinoma." Retrieved 2010-06-28.

[34] Rosai Juan,Breast In: Rosai and Ackerman's surgical pathology Volume-2, 10th Ed. Elsevier; 2012; 1689-1694.

[35] Orell SR, Sterrett GF, et al; Breat In: Orell and Sterret's Fine Needle Aspiration Cytology, 5th Ed. Elsevier; 2012; 188.

[36] Frost AR, Aksu A, Kurstin R, et al. Can nonproliferative breast disease and proliferative breast disease without atypia be distinguished by fine – needle aspiration cytology? *Cancer* 1997;81:22-8.

Chapter 5

Lobular Carcinoma In Situ

Lobular carcinoma in situ (LCIS) is usually diagnosed before menopause, most often between the ages of 40 & 50 years. Less than 10% of women diagnosed with LCIS have already gone through menopause. LCIS is extremely uncommon in men. Lobular carcinoma in situ (LCIS) is a condition caused by unusual cells in the lobules of the breast [1].

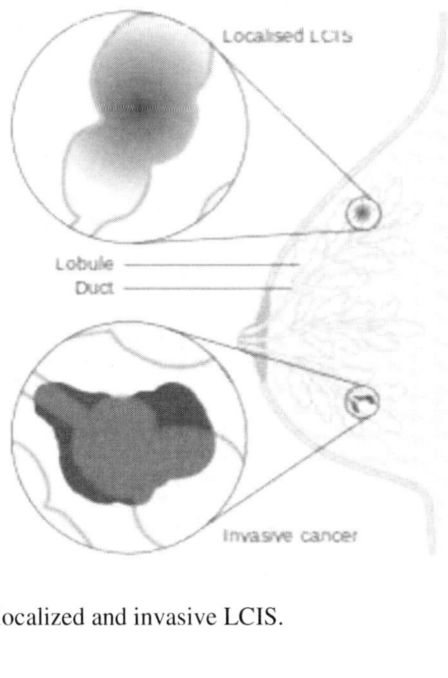

Figure 1. Showing localized and invasive LCIS.

Many do not considered it cancer, but it can indicate an increased risk of future cancer [2, 3, 4]. The national database registrars, however, consider it a malignancy [5].

Unlike ductal carcinoma in situ (DCIS), LCIS is not associated with calcification, and is typically an incidental finding in a biopsy performed for another reason. LCIS only accounts for about 15% of the in situ (ductal or lobular) breast cancers [6].

Genetics

Cells of LCIS and invasive lobular carcinoma have the same histology, appearing as single detached cells, as both have loss of expression of e-cadherin, the transmembrane protein mediating epithelial cell adhesion [7]. LCIS often have the same genetic alterations (such as loss of heterozygosity on chromosome 16q, the locus for the e-cadherin gene) as the adjacent area of invasive carcinoma [8].

Morphology

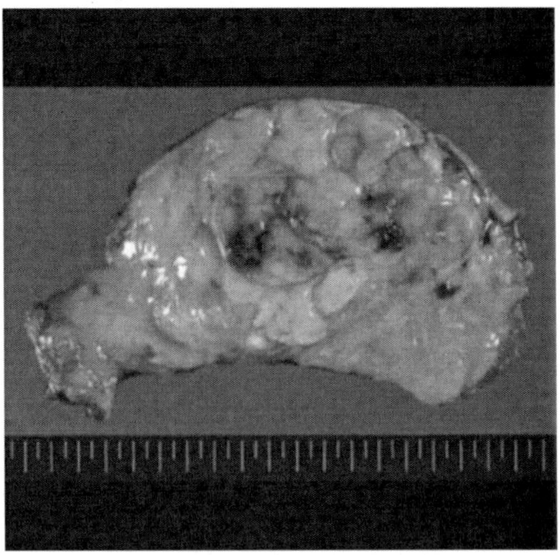

Figure 2. Gross Specimen showing lobular carcinoma in situ.

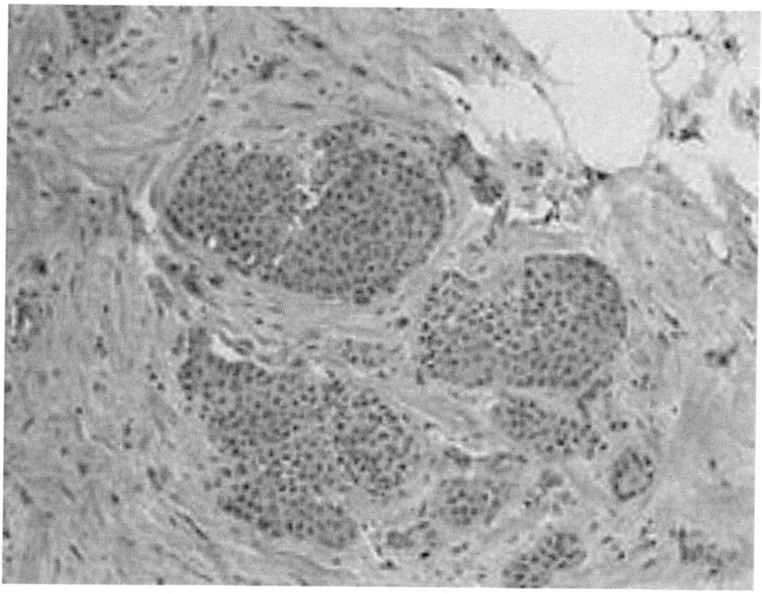

Figure 3. Microscopy of Lobular carcinoma in situ, H&E, 20x.

Table 1. Contrasting features of Atypical lobular hyperplasia and LCIS

	ALH	LCIS
Distention of acini	Less distended and distorted	Distended and distorted
Degree of involvement	Often only part of lobular unit	Major part of one or more lobular units
Luminal obliteration	Incomplete	Complete
Cellular composition	Less monotonous; may be variable cell types; less regularly spaced	Round, regular, monotonous; one cell type; evenly spaced
Cellular cohesion	More cohesive	No cohesive
Spread to ducts	Pagetoid spread may occur, but less well developed	Pagetoid spread and other forms

Like the cells of atypical lobular hyperplasia and invasive lobular carcinoma, the abnormal cells of LCIS consist of small cells with oval or round nuclei and small nucleoli detached from each other [9]. Mucin-containing signet-ring cells are commonly seen. LCIS generally leaves the underlying architecture intact and recognisable as lobules. Estrogen and progesterone receptors are present and HER2/neu overexpression is absent in most cases of LCIS [9]. 60% cases shows S100 positivity & scattered tumor cells shows positivity for mucin. It is distinguished from DCIS by lack of reactivity for E cadherin, B catenin and positivity for HMW keratin. Variant of LCIS include: Pleomorphic LCIS contain medium to large tumor cells with moderate to marked pleomorphism and occasional prominent nuclei with moderate to abundant cytoplasm. It shows mural and pagetoid pattern in which neighboring terminal duct cells form continuous row beneath the secretory epithelium [12].

Treatment Options

LCIS may be treated with close clinical follow-up and mammographic screening, tamoxifen or related hormone controlling drugs to reduce the risk of developing cancer, or bilateral prophylactic mastectomy. Some surgeons consider bilateral prophylactic mastectomy to be overly aggressive treatment except for certain high-risk cases [10].

Prognosis

LCIS (lobular neoplasia is considered pre-cancerous) is an indicator (marker) for identifying women with an increased risk of developing invasive breast cancer. This risk extends more than 20 years. Most of the risk relates to subsequent invasive ductal carcinoma rather than to invasive lobular carcinoma [10].

While older studies have shown that the increased risk is equal for both breasts, a more recent study suggests that the ipsilateral (same side) breast may be at greater risk [11].

References

[1] "Lobular Carcinoma in situ (LCIS)." *Breast Cancer*. Stanford Cancer Center.

[2] "Lobular carcinoma in situ: Marker for breast cancer risk." MayoClinic.com.

[3] "Breast Cancer Treatment." National Cancer Institute.

[4] Afonso N, Bouwman D (August 2008). "Lobular carcinoma in situ." *Eur. J. Cancer Prev.* 17 (4): 312–6. doi:10.1097/CEJ.0b013e3282f75e5d. PMID 18562954.

[5] Cancer, American Joint Committee on (2002). AJCC cancer staging handbook: from the AJCC cancer staging manual (6th ed.). New York: *Springer.* p. 260. ISBN 9780387952703.

[6] "Susan G. Komen for the Cure | Understanding Breast Cancer | Breast Facts | Statistics | Breast Cancer Statistics." Retrieved 2013-01-16.

[7] Hajra KM, Fearon ER (2002). "Cadherin and catenin alterations in human cancer." *Genes Chromosomes Cancer* 34 (3): 255–68. doi:10.1002/gcc.10083. PMID 12007186.

[8] Lakhani SR (2001). "Molecular genetics of solid tumors: translating research into clinical practice. What we could do now: breast cancer." *Mol Pathol* 54 (5): 281–4. doi:10.1136/mp.54.5.281. PMC 1187082. PMID 11577167.

[9] Cotran, Ramzi S.; Kumar, Vinay; Fausto, Nelson; Nelso Fausto; Robbins, Stanley L.; Abbas, Abul K. (2005). Robbins and Cotran pathologic basis of disease (7th ed.). St. Louis, MO: Elsevier Saunders. p. 1142. ISBN 0-7216-0187-1.

[10] "Breast Cancer Treatment (PDQ®) - National Cancer Institute - Lobular Carcinoma In Situ." Retrieved 2013-01-12.

[11] Page DL, Schuyler PA, DuPont WD, Jensen RA, Plummer WD Jr, Simpson JF (2003). "Atypical lobular hyperplasia as a unilateral predictor of breast cancer risk: a retrospective cohort study." *Lancet* 361 (9352): 125–9. doi:10.1016/S0140-6736(03)12230-1. PMID 12531579.

[12] Rosai Juan,Breast In: Rosai and Ackerman's surgical pathology Volume-2, 10th Ed. Elsevier; 2012; 1695.

Chapter 6

Invasive Ductal Carcinoma (IDC-NOS)

Tumors included in this category are all those in which stromal invasion is detectable, whether an in situ component is identifiable or not, and regardless of the relative proportion of the two components. In other words, it also includes so-called 'micro invasive carcinoma.' Like the in situ lesions, most of the invasive tumors can be divided into two major categories – ductal type and lobular type – acknowledging the existence of mixed and intermediate forms. It should be emphasized that the type of invasive carcinoma should be determined from its own appearance, rather than deduced from the type of in situ component present, if any, since there is not always correspondence between the two.

Cytoarchitectural Variants

The morphologic variations on the theme of invasive ductal carcinoma are innumerable. Some of them are distinctive enough to deserve recognition as special types, especially when associated with a particular behavior. The others, which represent approximately 75% of all cases, are generically designated as invasive ductal carcinomas of classic, ordinary, or not-otherwise-specified (NOS) type [1].

This lesion represents the prototypic expression of breast carcinoma and is the tumor type usually implied when the terms 'breast carcinoma' or 'breast cancer' are used without further qualification. The size, shape, consistency and type of margins are highly variable.

Grossly, the typical case is firm and poorly circumscribed, cuts with a resistant gritty sensation and shows a yellowish-gray cut surface, with trabeculae radiating through the surrounding parenchyma into the fat, resulting in the notorious stellate or crab-like configuration, from which the word 'cancer' has originated. Sometimes these strands are seen connecting with other tumor nodules located at some distance from the primary tumor. Areas of necrosis, hemorrhage, and cystic degeneration may be present, particularly in the larger neoplasms. The tumor may have invaded the overlying skin or the underlying fascia and pectoralis muscle. Tumors that are particularly hard because of the large amounts of stroma were traditionally referred to as 'scirrhous carcinomas' a term no longer used.

It is common for these neoplasms to exhibit 'chalky streaks' on the cut surface (Figure 1) a feature caused not by necrosis as generally believed, but by duct elastosis [681]. When this occurs, the appearance of the lesion has an uncanny resemblance to an unripe pear, further accentuated by the consistency and the sensation one has while cutting it.

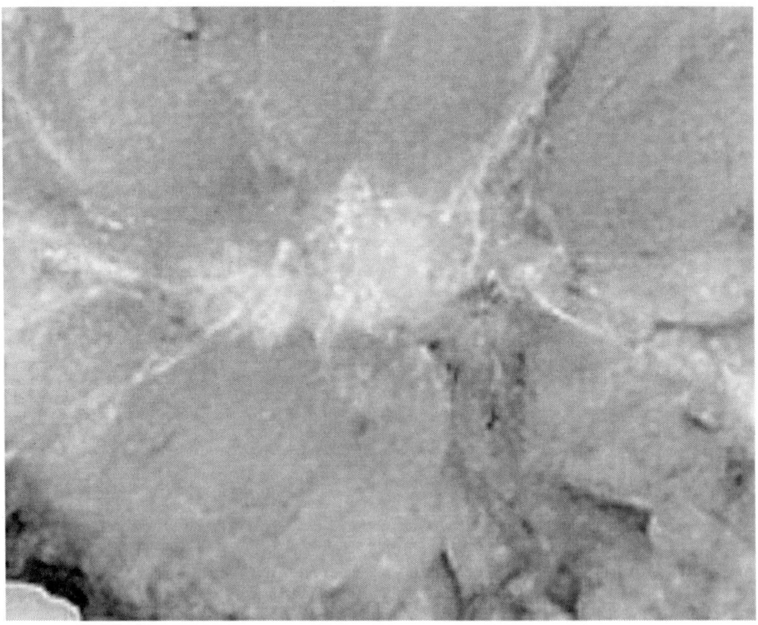

Figure 1. Showing chalky white appearance on the cut surface.

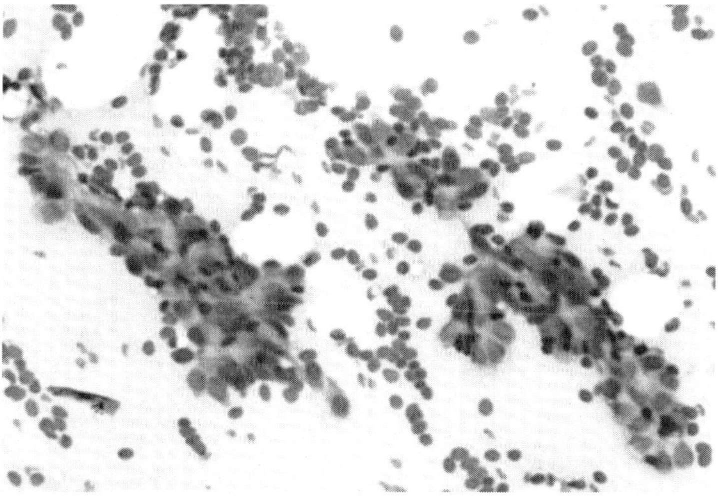

Figure 2. FNAC showing loose clusters of malignant ductal epithelial cells.

FNAC smears show moderately to highly cellular smear, single population of epithelial cells, no myoepithelial cells and no single bare bipolar nuclei. Variable loss of cell cohesion irregular clusters and spindle cells. Moderate to severe nuclear atypia, enlargement, pleomorphism, irregular nuclear membrane and chromatin (Figure 2).

Microscopically [2] the tumor can grow in diffuse sheets, well-defined nests, cords, or as individual cells (Figure 3). Glandular/tubular differentiation may be well developed, barely detectable, or altogether absent. Parenthetically, this is the reason why the term adenocarcinoma is not advisable as a synonym for invasive ductal carcinoma. The tumor cells vary in size and shape, but by definition they are larger and more pleomorphic than those of the classic form of invasive lobular carcinomas, their nuclei and nucleoli are more prominent, and mitotic figures are more numerous. Areas of necrosis occur in approximately 60% of cases [3]. Foci of squamous metaplasia, apocrine metaplasia, or clear cell changes may be seen. The amount of stroma ranges from none to abundant and its appearance from densely fibrotic to cellular (desmoplastic). In cases with abundant stroma, it may be difficult to identify the tumor cells. Bulky masses of elastic tissue are present in approximately 90% of cases. As already indicated, this 'elastosis' which can involve the wall of the ducts and the vessels (mainly veins), is responsible for the chalky streaks seen on gross examination [4]. Calcification can be detected in approximately 60% of cases, either as coarse or fine granules or, rarely, as psammoma bodies [5]. A mononuclear inflammatory infiltrate of variable intensity is usually present at the interphase between tumor and stroma. Granulomatous inflammation is rarely seen [6].

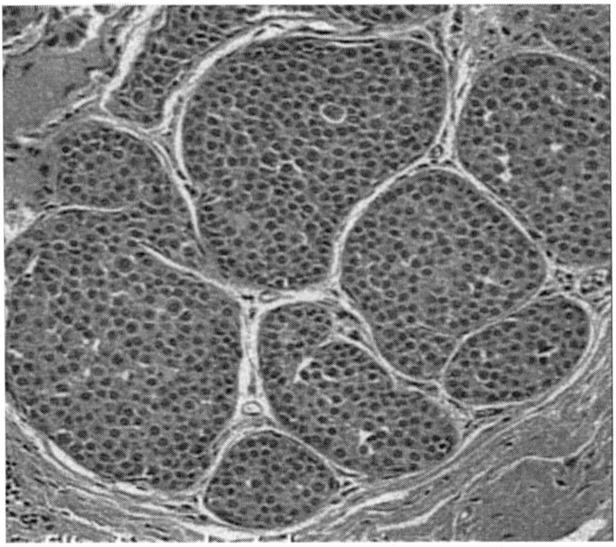

Figure 3. Microscopic of IDC shows tumor cell in diffuse sheets and clusters.

IHC shows immunoreactivity for EMA and HMW Keratin (Figure 4).

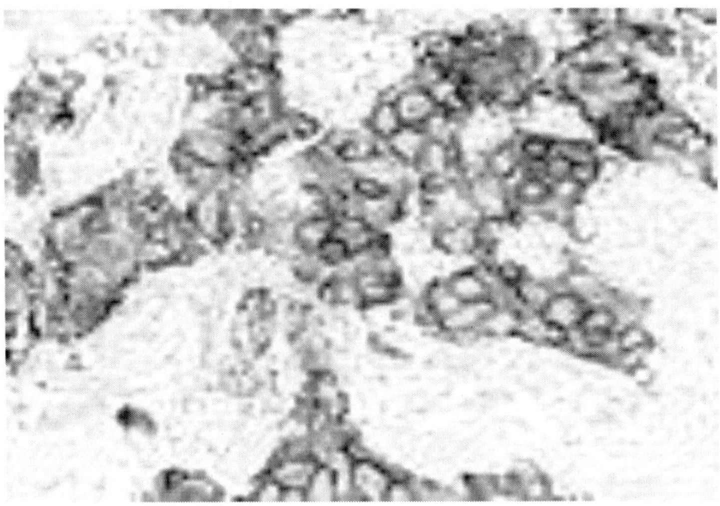

Figure 4. IHC showing positivity for EMA.

Variants include:

1) **Tubular carcinoma:-** Well differentiated carcinoma with average age of 50 years. Grossly shows poorly circumscribed margins with hard consistency (Figure 5). Tumor is small with mean diameter of 1cm. Microscopically,it shows characteristic angulated shape of the glands and cellular stroma (Figure 6). Glands having open lumina with basophilic secretion. Apocrine type of snouts in the apical cytoplasm. Formation of trabecular bars and lack of myoepithelial cell component.

Metastasis to axillary nodes occurs in 10% of cases and prognosis is excellent.

Sometimes, a tubular carcinoma pattern is seen in association with an ordinary invasive ductal carcinoma. The prognosis of these 'mixed' tumors is substantially worse than for pure tubular carcinoma [7, 8, 9].

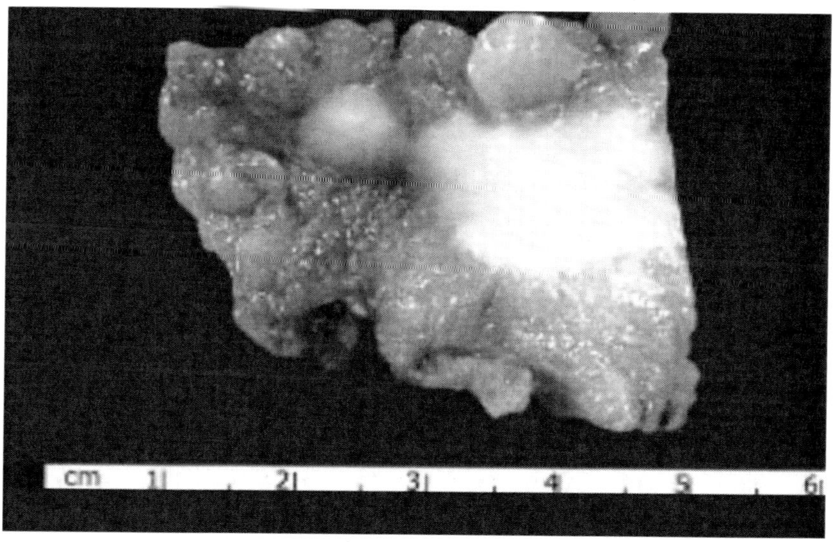

Figure 5. Gross picture shows poorly circumscribed margine with hard consistency.

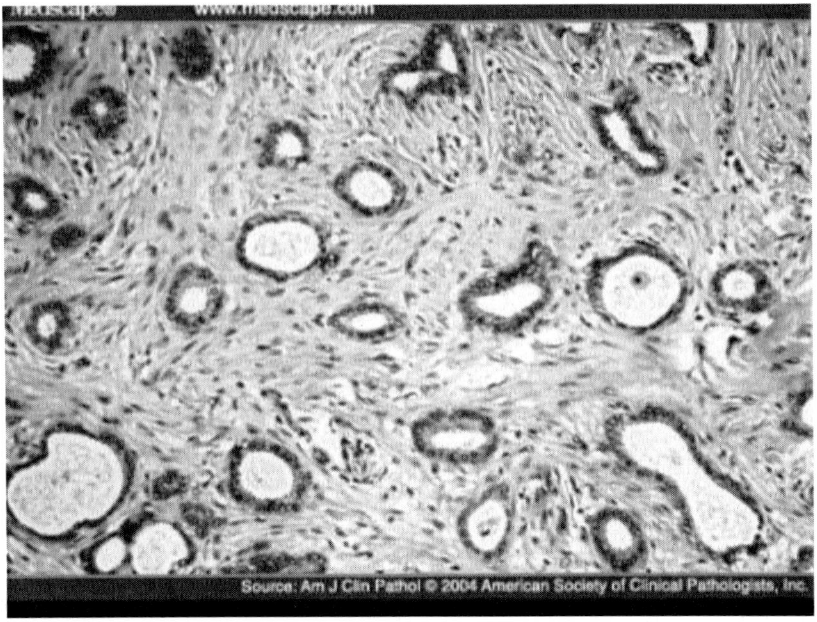

Figure 6. Tubular carcinoma shows angulated gland in cellular stroma.

2) **Cribriform carcinoma:-** It is a rare form of breast malignancy closely related to tubular carcinoma with an excellent prognosis. The tumor has a cribriform appearance and stromal invasion (Figures 7 and 8).

3) **Mucinous carcinoma (Mucoid/Colloid/Gelatinous carcinoma):-** Usually occurs in postmenopausal women. Grossly it is well circumscribed, crepitant to palpation and formed by currant Jelly like mass (Figure 9). Microscopically, the classic and often quoted description is that of small clusters of tumor cells ‘floating in a sea of mucin.’ These clusters may be solid, exhibit acinar formations, or form micropapillarystructures (Figure 10) [10]. The mucin is almost entirely extracellular, and it may be of acid or neutral type [11].

Pure mucinous carcinoma is associated with a very low incidence (2–4%) of nodal metastases [12, 13, 14]. Consequently, the pure form of mucinous carcinoma carries an excellent short-term prognosis, particularly when the tumor measures less than 3 cm (or even less than 5 cm) in diameter [15, 13].

A further variation on the theme is represented by *mucinous cystadenocarcinoma*, an exceptionally rare tumor composed predominantly of tall columnar cells with abundant intracytoplasmic mucin and a multicystic gross quality similar to that of its ovarian counterpart [16, 17, and 18].

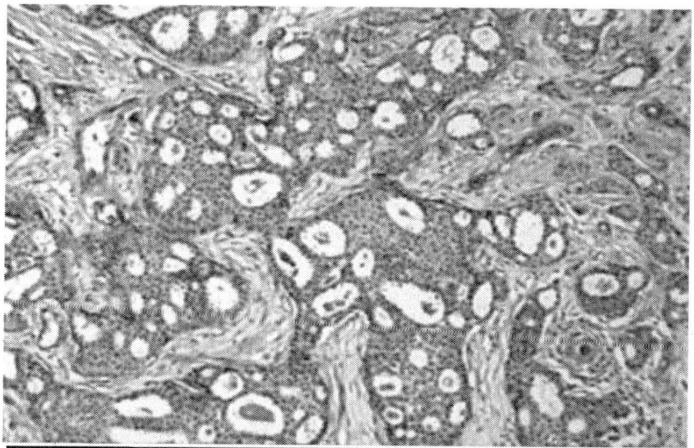

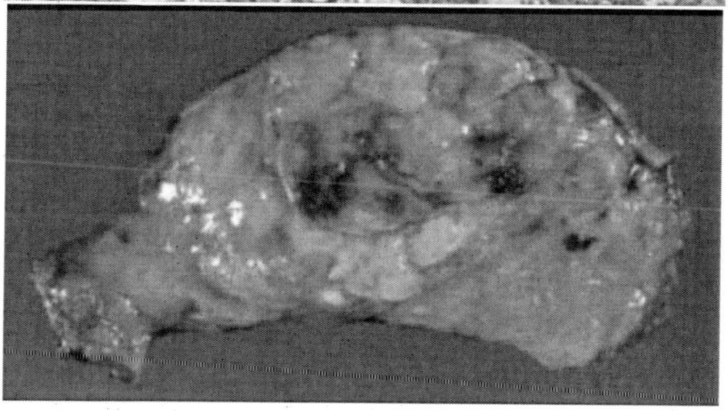

Figures 7 and 8. Microscopic picture showing cribriform pattern and Gross appearance of cribriform carcinoma.

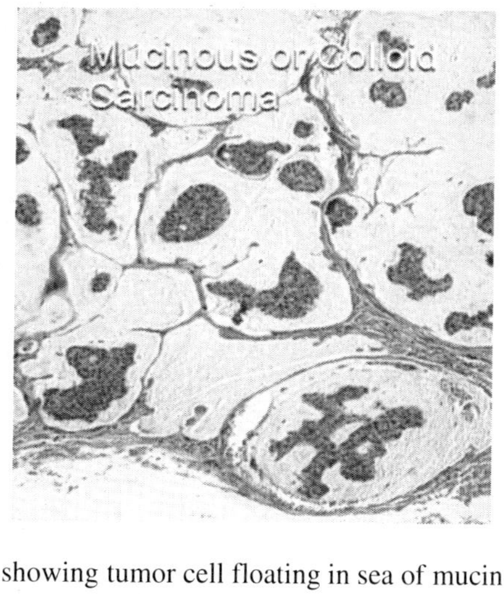

Figure 9. Microscopy showing tumor cell floating in sea of mucin.

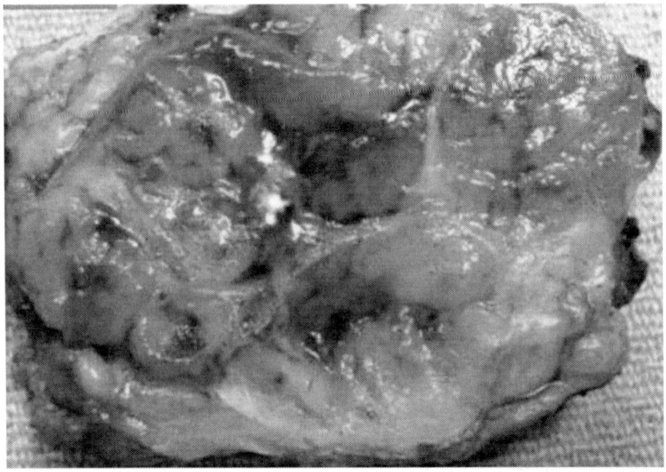

Figure 10. Gross showing currant jelly like mass.

5) Invasive papillary carcinoma:- The invasive component of a papillary carcinoma may also be papillary or have the features of an ordinary ductal-type carcinoma (Figure 11), the prognosis is substantially better for the former [19]. This tumor is said to occur more frequently among whites and postmenopausal women, [20] but, on the whole, it remains a very rare entity.

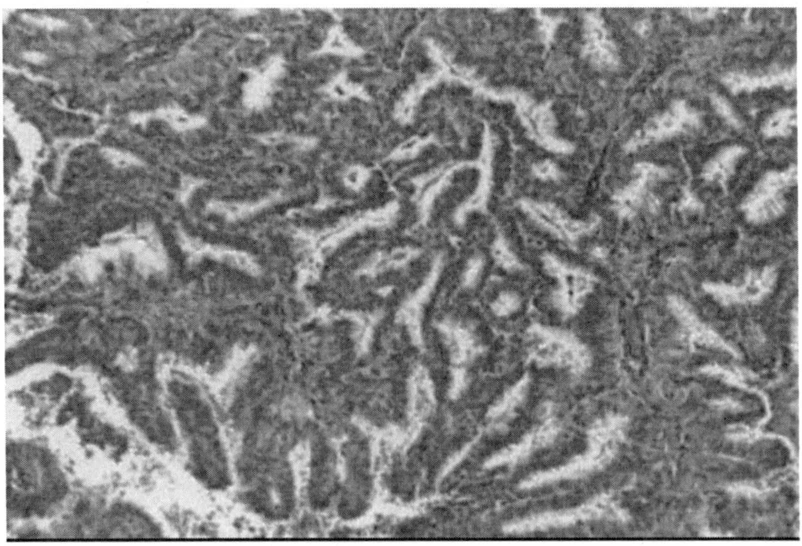

Figure 11. Showing papillae formations of malignant ductal epithelial cells.

6) **Invasive micropapillary carcinoma:-** Microscopically, it bears a close similarity with micropapillary carcinoma of other organs, notably endometrium, ovary, and bladder [21]. It is a highly invasive tumor characterized by the formation of pseudopapillary structures lacking a fibrovascular core and by tubular structures free-floating in clear empty spaces (Figure 12). The nuclear grade is typically high [22]. Psammoma bodies are present in about one half of the cases [23]. Immunohistochemically, is usually positive for estrogen receptors and mammaglobin, and negative for PAX8 and WT1 [24–25]. Lymph node metastasis is the rule (it's frequency being directly related to the presence of lymph vessel permeation [26], local recurrence is high, and the survival rate is distinctly lower than for conventional invasive ductal carcinoma [27, 28].

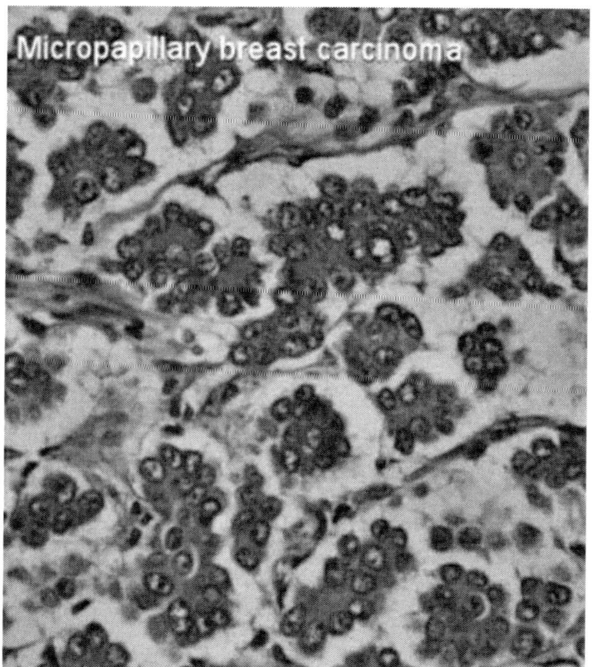

Figure 12. Showing micropapillae formations.

7) **Apocrine carcinoma:-** Apocrine carcinoma is a very rare form of breast malignancy (ranging from 1% to 4% of all cases). Composed entirely or predominantly of apocrine-type epithelium [29, 30]. The large tumor cells have an abundant acidophilic, somewhat granular cytoplasm, which may

contain eosinophilic or golden brown granules that are strongly PAS positive. The nuclei are vesicular and nucleoli are prominent. Glandular differentiation is usually found, the luminal portion of the tumor having a characteristic bulbous expansion (apocrine snout) (Figure 13). Since apocrine changes in the breast are usually indicative of benignancy (even when the cells exhibit prominent nucleolar enlargement), and the diagnosis of apocrine carcinoma should be made only when the architectural features are clearly those of a malignant tumor. It is also important to limit the diagnosis of apocrine carcinoma to malignant tumors in which the apocrine change is widespread, in view of the fact that focal apocrine differentiation (as detected by GCDFP-15) can be detected in close to 10% of ordinary carcinomas [31].

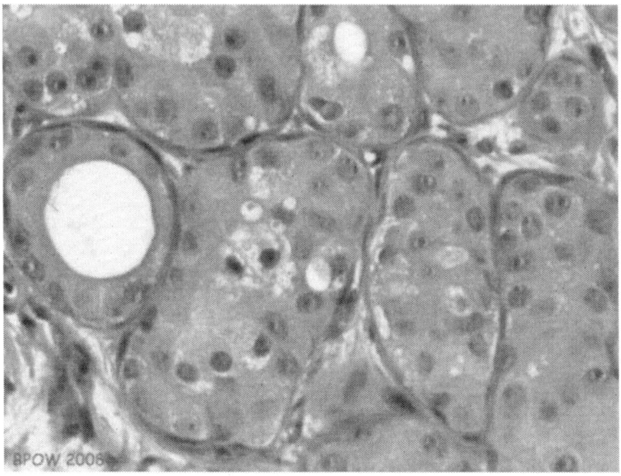

Figure 13. Showing malignant oncocytic cells.

8) **Secretary (juvenile) carcinoma:-** This rare form of breast carcinoma is seen primarily in children, but it can also occur in adults [32, 34, and 36]. Grossly, it is well circumscribed and usually small. The microscopic appearance is distinctive. The margins are of the 'pushing' type, and prominent hyalinization is often present in the central portion (Figure 14). The microscopic appearance is distinctive. Tubuloalveolar and focally papillary formations lined by cells with a vacuolated (sometimes hypernephroid) cytoplasm is seen forming Lumina filled by an eosinophilic PAS-positive secretion [33, 35, and 36]. Nucleoli may be prominent, but mitoses are very scanty. The overall prognosis is excellent, most series quoting a 5-year

survival rate close to 100% [33]. Local recurrences and nodal metastases can develop, sometimes very late in the course of the disease [32, 35, and 36].

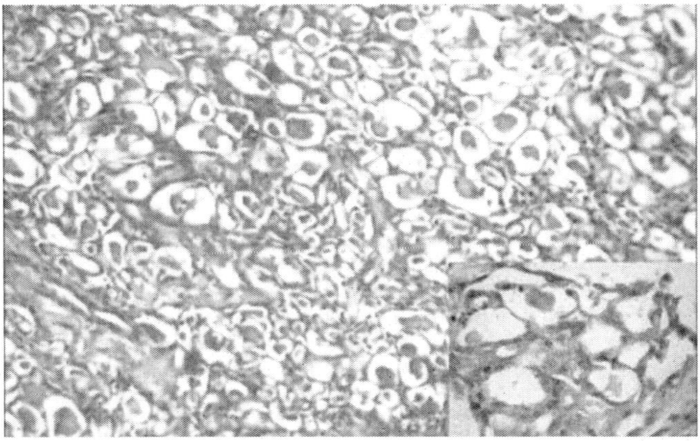

Figure 14. Microscopic appearance showing secretary Carcinoma.

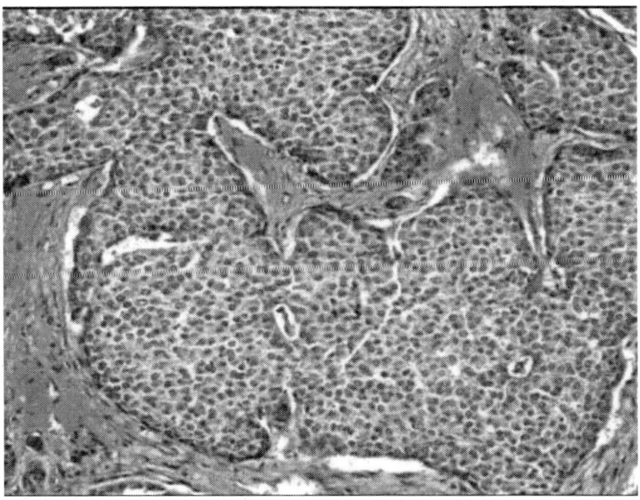

Figure 15. Carcinoid tumor showing neuroendocrine cells *i*n nests, islands.

9) Carcinomas with neuroendocrine features (including so-called 'carcinoid tumor')-The term carcinoid tumor was originally proposed for a type of invasive ductal carcinoma exhibiting features consistent with neuroendocrine differentiation [38]. Multicentricity and bilaterality can occur [38]. There are no distinctive gross features. Microscopically, the tumor cells are small, arranged in solid nests separated by fibrous tissue (Figure 15).

Ribbons and rosette like formations may be seen. Mitoses are generally rare. The presence of an intraductal component and of mucin secretion has been detected in a minority of the cases [38]. The microscopic differential diagnosis includes lobular carcinoma and a metastasis to the breast of a carcinoid tumor located elsewhere. The immunohistochemical positivity that has been obtained for chromogranin, synaptophysin, and NSE [37, 40, 42, 43] and in some instances for specific hormone peptides [39, 41].

Spread-Related Variants

1) Inflammatory carcinoma- The term inflammatory carcinoma was originally used in a clinical context for a type of breast carcinoma in which the entire breast was reddened and warm, with widespread edema of the skin, thus simulating the appearance of mastitis [50].

Pathologic studies in some of those cases revealed the lesion to be an undifferentiated carcinoma with widespread carcinomatosis of the dermal lymphatic vessels. Patients may have inflammatory carcinoma clinically in the absence of dermal invasion; conversely, widespread permeation of dermal lymphatics can be seen in the absence of the clinical features of inflammatory carcinoma (so-called 'occult' inflammatory carcinoma) [50] (Figure 16). From a prognostic standpoint, the presence of dermal lymphatic permeation on microscopic examination is a sign of ominous prognosis, whether the clinical appearance is that of an inflammatory carcinoma or not [50, 51].

2) Paget disease- Paget disease is the name given to a crusted lesion of the nipple caused by breast carcinoma, as originally described by Sir James Paget in 1874 [52]. It is accompanied in nearly all instances by an underlying breast carcinoma of in situ ductal type, with or without associated stromal invasion. The management and prognosis depend largely on the intraductal versus invasive nature of the underlying carcinoma and on the presence or absence of axillary lymph node involvement. Clinically, these weeping, eczema-like lesions are centered in the nipple. Later they may involve the areola and surrounding epidermis, but they rarely extend more than a few centimeters.

Microscopically, large clear cells with atypical nuclei are seen within the epidermis, usually concentrated along the basal layer but also permeating the malpighian layer. The cells can be isolated or in clusters, and sometimes they form small glandular structures (Figure 17) [52]. Occasionally, intracytoplasmic melanin granules are present, a feature that may result in a mistaken diagnosis of malignant melanoma; these granules have probably been transferred from neighboring melanocytes by the process of cytocrinia [52, 53].

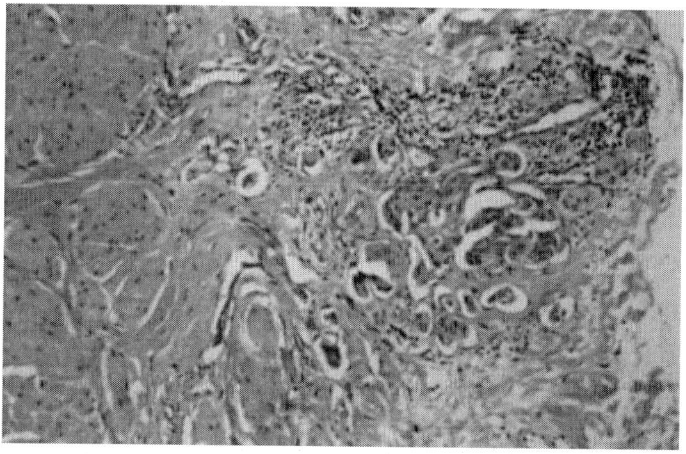

Figure 16. Microscopic appearance of inflammatory carcinoma.

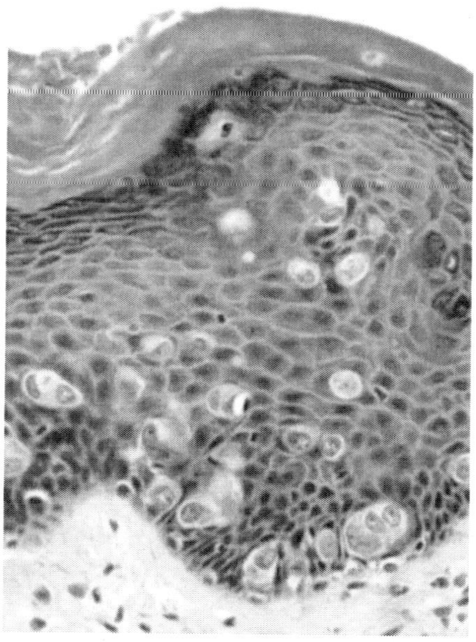

Figure 17. Showing Paget's disease shows large clear cell within the basal layer of epidermis.

References

[1] Berg JW, Hutter RV: Breast cancer. *Cancer* 1995; 75:257-269.

[2] Fisher ER, Gregorio RM: Fisher B, with the assistance of Redmond C, Vellios F, Sommers SC, and cooperating investigators. The pathology of invasive breast cancer. A syllabus derived from findings of the National Surgical Adjuvant Breast Project (Protocol No. 4). *Cancer* 1975; 36:1-85.

[3] 676. Fisher ER, Palekar AS, Gregorio RM, Redmond C, Fisher B: Pathological findings from the National Surgical Adjuvant Breast Project (Protocol No. 4). IV. Significance of tumor necrosis. *Hum Pathol* 1978; 9:523-530.

[4] Azzopardi JG, Laurini RN: Elastosis in breast cancer. *Cancer* 1974; 33:174-183.

[5] Fisher ER, Gregorio RM: Fisher B, with the assistance of Redmond C, Vellios F, Sommers SC, and cooperating investigators. The pathology of invasive breast cancer. A syllabus derived from findings of the National Surgical Adjuvant Breast Project (Protocol No. 4). *Cancer* 1975; 36:1-85.

[6] Oberman HA: Invasive carcinoma of the breast with granulomatous response. *Am J ClinPathol* 1987; 88:718-721.

[7] Carstens PHB, Greenberg RA, Francis D, Lyon H: Tubular carcinoma of the breast. A long term follow-up. *Histopathology* 1985; 9:271-280.

[8] Deos PH, Norris HJ: Well-differentiated (tubular) carcinoma of the breast. A clinicopathologic study of 145 pure and mixed cases. *Am J ClinPathol* 1982; 78:1-7.

[9] Parl FF, Richardson LD: The histologic and biologic spectrum of tubular carcinoma of the breast. *Hum Pathol* 1983; 14:694-698.

[10] Bal A, Joshi K, Sharma SC, Das A, Verma A, Wig JD: Prognostic significance of micropapillary pattern in pure mucinous carcinoma of the breast. *Int J SurgPathol* 2008; 16:251-256.

[11] Walker RA: Mucoid carcinomas of the breast. A study using mucinhistochemistry and peanut lectin. *Histopathology* 1982; 6:571-579.

[12] Diab SG, Clark GM, Osborne CK, Libby A, Allred DC, Elledge RM: Tumor characteristics and clinical outcome of tubular and mucinous breast carcinomas. *J ClinOncol* 1999; 17:1442-1448.

[13] Norris HJ, Taylor HB: Prognosis of mucinous (gelatinous) carcinoma of the breast. *Cancer* 1965; 18:879-885754.

[14] Rasmussen BB, Rose C, Christensen IB: Prognostic factors in primary mucinous breast carcinoma. *Am J ClinPathol* 1987; 87:155-160. 737.

[15] Clayton F: Pure mucinous carcinomas of breast. Morphologic features and prognostic correlates. *Hum Pathol* 1986; 17:34-38.

[16] Coyne JD, Irion L: Mammary mucinous cystadenocarcinoma. *Histopathology* 2006; 49:659-660.

[17] Koenig C, Tavassoli FA: Mucinous cystadenocarcinoma of the breast. *Am J SurgPathol* 1998; 22:698-703.

[18] Nassar H, Qureshi H, Volkanadsay N, Visscher D: Clinicopathologic analysis of solid papillary carcinoma of the breast and associated invasive carcinomas. *Am J SurgPathol* 2006; 30:501-5.

[19] Fisher ER, Palekar AS, Redmond C, Barton B, Fisher B: Pathologic findings from the National Surgical Adjuvant Breast Project (Protocol No. 4). VI. Invasive papillary cancer. *Am J ClinPathol* 1980; 73:313-322.

[20] Moritani S, Ichihara S, Hasegawa M, Endo T, Oiwa M, Yoshikawa K, Sato Y, Aoyama H, Hayashi T, Kushima R: Serous papillary adenocarcinoma of the female genital organs and invasive micropapillary carcinoma of the breast. Are WT1, CA125, and GCDFP-15 useful in differential diagnosis?. *Hum Pathol* 2008; 39:666-671.

[21] DelaCruz C, Moriya T, Endoh M, Watanabe M, Takeyama J, Yang M, Oguma M, Sakamoto K, Suzuki T, Hirakawa H, Orita Y, Ohuchi N, Sasano H: Invasive micropapillary carcinoma of the breast: clinicopathological and immunohistochemical study. *PatholInt* 2004; 54:90-96.

[22] Pettinato G, Manivel CJ, Panico L, Sparano L, Petrella G: Invasive micropapillary carcinoma of the breast: clinicopathologic study of 62 cases of a poorly recognized variant with highly aggressive behavior. *Am J ClinPathol* 2004; 121:857-866.

[23] Kuroda N, Sugimoto T, Takahashi T, Moriki T, Toi M, Miyazaki E, Hiroi M, Enzan H: Invasive micropapillary carcinoma of the breast: an immunohistochemical study of neoplastic and stromal cells. *Int J SurgPathol* 2005; 13:51-55.

[24] DelaCruz C, Moriya T, Endoh M, Watanabe M, Takeyama J, Yang M, Oguma M, Sakamoto K, Suzuki T, Hirakawa H, Orita Y, Ohuchi N, Sasano H: Invasive micropapillary carcinoma of the breast: clinicopathological and immunohistochemical study. *PatholInt* 2004; 54:90-96.

[25] Acs G, Esposito NN, Rakosy Z, Laronga C, Zhang PJ: Invasive ductal carcinomas of the breast showing partial reversed cell polarity are associated with lymphatic tumor spread and may represent part of a spectrum of invasive micropapillary carcinoma. *Am J Surg Pathol* 2010; 34:1637-1646.

[26] Acs G, Paragh G, Chuang ST, Laronga C, Zhang PJ: The presence of micropapillary features and retraction artifact in core needle biopsy material predicts lymph node metastasis in breast carcinoma. *Am J SurgPathol* 2009; 33:202-210.

[27] Chen L, Fan Y, Lang RG, Guo XJ, Sun YL, Cui LF, Liu FF, Wei J, Zhang XM, Fu L: Breast carcinoma with micropapillary features: clinicopathologic study and long-term follow-up of 100 cases. *Int J SurgPathol* 2008; 16:155-163.

[28] Pettinato G, Manivel CJ, Panico L, Sparano L, Petrella G: Invasive micropapillary carcinoma of the breast: clinicopathologic study of 62 cases of a poorly recognized variant with highly aggressive behavior. *Am J ClinPathol* 2004; 121:857-866.

[29] Abati AD, Kimmel M, Rosen PP: Apocrine mammary carcinoma. A clinicopathologic study of 72 cases. *Am J Clin Pathol* 1990; 94:371-377.

[30] O'Malley FP, Bane A: An update on apocrine lesions of the breast. *Histopathology* 2008; 52:3-10.

[31] Eusebi V, Millis RR, Cattani MG, Bussolati G, Azzopardi JG: Apocrine carcinoma of the breast. A morphologic and immunocytochemical study. *Am J Pathol* 1986; 123:532-541.

[32] Krausz T, Jenkins D, Grontoft O, Pollock DJ, Azzopardi JG: Secretory carcinoma of the breast in adults. Emphasis on late recurrence and metastasis. *Histopathology* 1989; 14:25-36.

[33] McDivitt RW, Stewart FW: Breast carcinoma in children. *JAMA* 1966; 195:388-390.

[34] Oberman HA: Secretory carcinoma of the breast in adults. *Am J SurgPathol* 1980; 4:465-470.

[35] Rosen PP, Cranor ML: Secretory carcinoma of the breast. *Arch Pathol Lab Med* 1991; 115:141-144.

[36] Tavassoli FA, Norris HJ: Secretory carcinoma of the breast. *Cancer* 1980; 45:2404-2413.

[37] Bussolati G, Papotti M, Sapino A, Gugliotta P, Ghiringhello B, Azzopardi JG: Endocrine markers in argyrophilic carcinomas of the breast. *Am J SurgPathol* 1987; 11:248-256.

[38] Cubilla AL, Woodruff JM: Primary carcinoid tumor of the breast. A report of eight patients. *Am J SurgPathol* 1977; 1:283-292.

[39] Nesland JM, Memoli VA, Holm R, Gould VE, Johannessen JV: Breast carcinomas with neuroendocrine differentiation. *Ultrastruct Pathol* 1985; 8:225-240.

[40] Pagani A, Papotti M, Hofler H, Weiler R, Winkler H, Bussolati G: Chromogranin A and B gene expression in carcinomas of the breast. Correlation of immunocytochemical, immunoblot, and hybridization analyses. *Am J Pathol* 1990; 136:319-327.

[41] Scopsi L, Balslev E, Brunner N, Poulsen HS, Andersen J, Rank F, Larsson LI: Immunoreactive opioid peptides in human breast cancer. *Am J Pathol* 1989; 134:473-479.

[42] Uccini S, Monardo F, Paradiso P, Masciangelo R, Marzullo A, Ruco LP, Baroni CD: Synaptophysin in human breast carcinomas. *Histopathology* 1991; 18:271-273.

[43] 866. Wilander E, Páhlman S, Sällström J, Lindgren A: Neuron-specific enolase expression and neuroendocrine differentiation in carcinomas of the breast. *Arch Pathol Lab Med* 1987; 111:830-832.

[44] Bauer TW, Rostock RA, Eggleston JC, Baral E: Spindle cell carcinoma of the breast. Four cases and review of the literature. *Hum Pathol* 1984; 15:147-152.

[45] Drudis T, Arroyo C, Van Hoeven K, Cordon-Cardo C, Rosen PP: The pathology of low-grade adenosquamous carcinoma of the breast. An immunohistochemical study. *Pathol Annu* 1994; 29(Pt 2):181-197.

[46] 922. Eusebi V, Lamovec J, Cattani MG, Fedeli F, Millis RR: Acantholytic variant of squamous-cell carcinoma of the breast. *Am J Surg Pathol* 1986; 10:855-861.

[47] Foschini MP, Fulcheri E, Baraechini P, Ceccarelli C, Betts CM, Eusebi V: Squamous cell carcinoma with prominent myxoidstroma. *Hum Pathol* 1990; 21:859-865.

[48] Gersell DJ, Katzenstein A-LA: Spindle cell carcinoma of the breast. A clinicopathologic and ultrastructural study. *Hum Pathol* 1981; 12:550-561.

[49] Ho BC, Tan HW, Lee VK, Tan PH: Preoperative and intraoperative diagnosis of low-grade adenosquamous carcinoma of the breast: potential diagnostic pitfalls. *Histopathology* 2006; 49:603-611.

[50] Buzdar AU, Montague ED, Barker JL, Hortobagyi GN, Blumenschein GR: Management of inflammatory carcinoma of breast with combined modality approach. An update. *Cancer* 1981; 47:2537-2542.

[51] Chang S, Parker SL, Pham T, Buzdar AU, Hursting SD: Inflammatory breast carcinoma incidence and survival: the surveillance, epidemiology, and end results program of the National Cancer Institute, 1975–1992. *Cancer* 1998; 82:2366-2372.

[52] Ashikari R, Park K, Huvos AG, Urban JA: Paget's disease of the breast. *Cancer* 1970; 26:680-685.

[53] Azzopardi JG, Eusebi V: Melanocyte colonization and pigmentation of breast carcinoma. *Histopathology* 1977; 1:21-30.

Chapter 7

Invasive Lobular Carcinoma

Invasive lobular carcinoma accounts for 5-10% of invasive breast cancer [1, 2].

Grossly the tumor is fixed to the surrounding tissue with concave cut face. The tumor is hard, gritty ('unripe pear'), color is variable often streaked with yellow (elastic tissue).

Microscopically it is characterized by presence of small and uniform tumor cells growing singly in Indian file pattern, concentric fashion around lobules. It has abundant stroma of dense fibrous type. Contain foci of periductal and perivenous elastosis [8].

FNAC shows cells single and in small clusters, single file is the characteristic feature. The cytological features are scanty cytoplasm, small naked hyperchromatic nuclei intracytoplasmic mucin /signet ring cell seen with thick eosinophilic background.

Histological Variants include:-

1) Classic type: - The malignant cells lack cohesion and are arranged individually or in a linear manner (Indian files), or as narrow trabeculae within the stroma. The lack of cohesion in these tumors is particularly distinctive. A "targetoid" arrangement is often present around residual normal mammary structures. The persistence of normal glandular structures is often evident within lobular carcinomas, whereas it is rare in ductal tumors. "Skip areas," i.e., foci of infiltrating carcinoma separated by areas of uninvolved mammary tissue- are common feature of lobular carcinoma. Necrosis is rarely, if ever,

present. Intracellular mucin is frequent. Although the classical "bulls eye" appearance of intracytoplasmic lumina seen with the combined alcian blue/PAS stain is said to be typical of lobular carcinoma, both in situ and invasive. (Figure 1) [10].

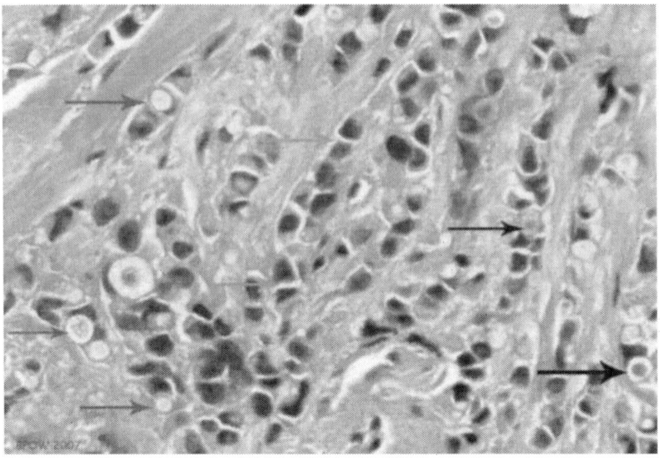

Figure 1. Classical type showing Indian file pattern.

2) Alveolar Type: - When the sheets of cells are smaller and arranged in rounded aggregates, the pattern has been termed "alveolar" and indeed it may be difficult to distinguish this from in situ lobular carcinoma (Figure 2) [11].

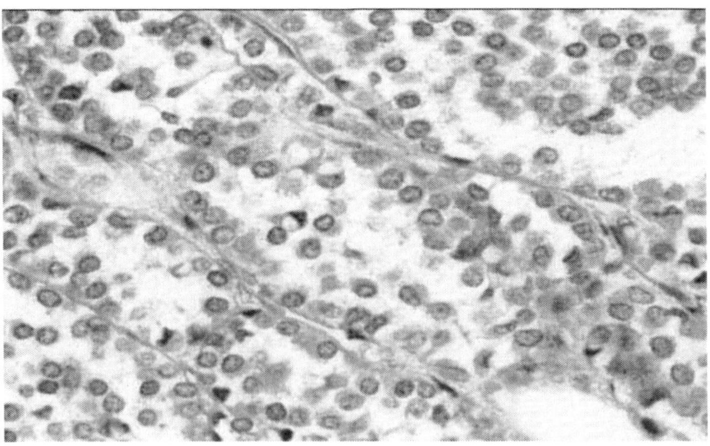

Figure 2. Alveolar type smaller sheets of cells arranged in rounded aggregates.

3) Solid type: - The malignant cells grow in sheets that engulf normal structures and infiltrate the fat in a growth pattern similar to that seen in lymphoma. (Figure 3) [11].

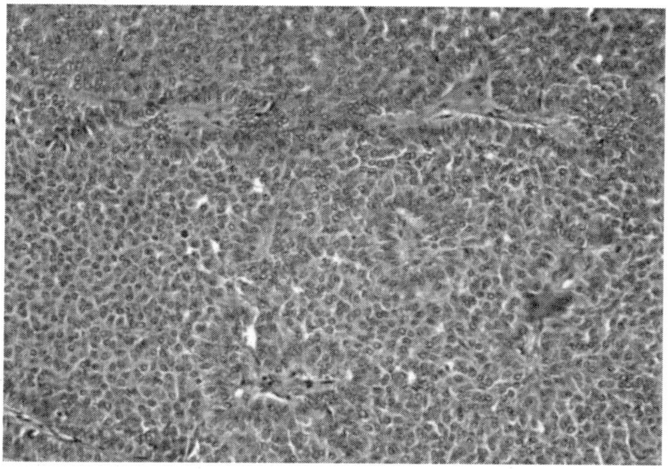

Figure 3. Solid type cells in sheets.

4) Tubulolobular type:-Occasionally, the cells form tubules but these are usually small and poorly developed. The term tubulolobular has also been used to describe carcinomas with a mixed pattern of typical tubular and typical lobular carcinoma (Figure 4) [12].

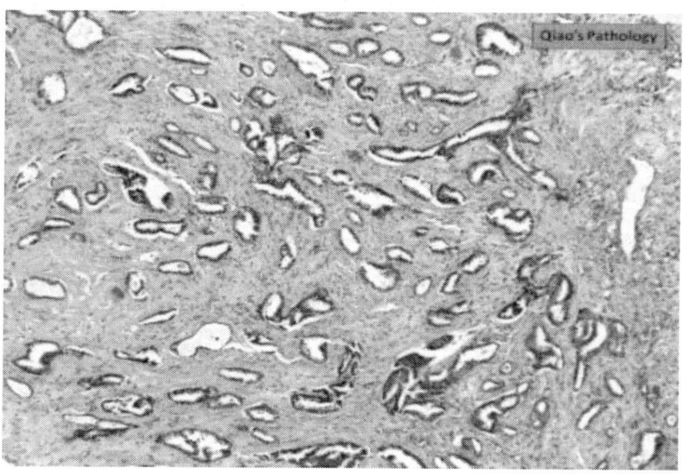

Figure 4. Tubulolobular type cells in tubules and lobular arranged.

5) Pleomorphic type: - The cells are more pleomorphic, sometimes with apocrine or histiocytoid features. The typical pattern of infiltration and lack of cellular cohesion, however, indicates that these lesions arc of lobular type (Figure 5) [13, 14, 15].

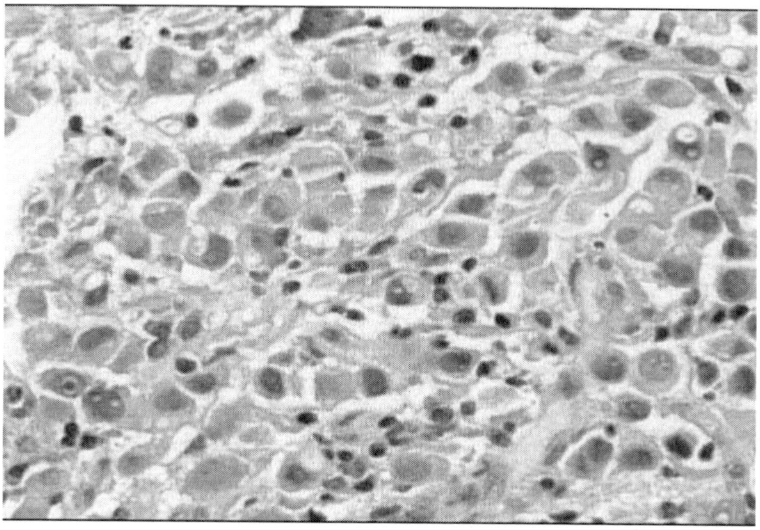

Figure 5. Pleomorphic type of invasive lobular carcinoma.

6) Mixed type: - Shows mixed pattern (Figure 6)

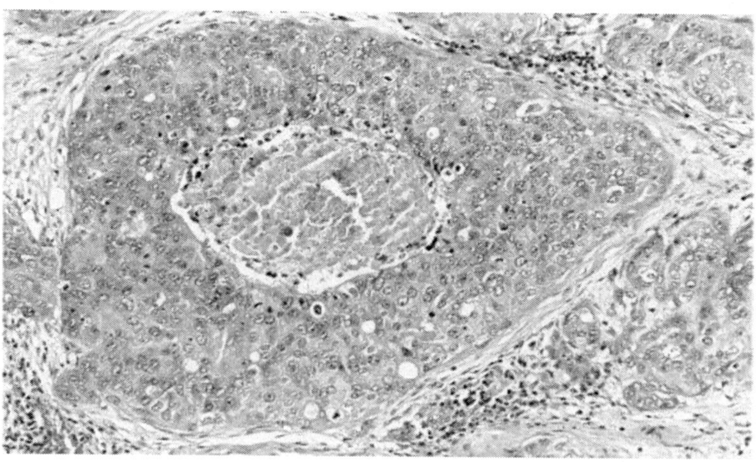

Figure 6. Mixed type.

Overall, the five-year survival rate of invasive lobular carcinoma was approximately 85% in 2003 [6].

Immunohistochemistry

Classic ILC typically express estrogen and progesterone receptors and rarely show overexpression of the HER2/neu protein or accumulation of the p53 gene product.

Loss of E-cadherin is common in lobular carcinoma but is also seen in other breast cancers [7].

IHC also shows HMW keratin positivity.

Genetic basis for loss of E cadherin CDH1 genes.

Differential diagnosis includes: - 1) IDC (Infiltrating Ductal Carcinoma): - distinguished by small size and uniformity of the cell and their lack of cohesiveness 2) Carcinoma with neuroendocrine features 3) Malignant lymphoma 4) Malignant histiocytosis [8].

References

[1] Pointon KS, Cunningham DA (August 1999). "Ultrasound findings in pure invasive lobular carcinoma of the breast: comparison with matched cases of invasive ductal carcinoma of the breast." *Breast* 8 (4): 188–90. doi:10.1054/brst.1999.0042. PMID 14731438.

[2] Boughey JC, Wagner J, Garrett BJ, et al. (March 2009). "Neoadjuvant Chemotherapy in Invasive Lobular Carcinoma May Not Improve Rates of Breast Conservation." *Ann. Surg. Oncol.* 16 (6): 1606–11. doi:10.1245/s10434-009-0402-z. PMID 19280264.

[3] Moore MM, Borossa G, Imbrie JZ, et al. (June 2000). "Association of Infiltrating Lobular Carcinoma With Positive Surgical Margins After Breast-Conservation Therapy." *Ann. Surg.* 231 (6): 877–82. doi:10.1097/00000658-200006000-00012.PMC 1421077. PMID 10816631.

[4] Spencer JT, Shutter J (March 2009). "Synchronous bilateral invasive lobular breast cancer presenting as carcinomatosis in a male." *Am. J. Surg. Pathol.* 33 (3): 470–4. doi:10.1097/PAS.0b013e318190d10d. PMID 19092630.

[5] Fletcher's diagnostic histopathology of tumors. 3rd Ed. p. 931-932.

[6] Arpino G, Bardou VJ, Clark GM, Elledge RM (2004). "Infiltrating lobular carcinoma of the breast: tumor characteristics and clinical outcome." *Breast Cancer Res.* 6 (3): R149–56. doi:10.1186/bcr767. PMC 400666. PMID 15084238.

[7] Varga Z, Mallon E. (Oct 2009). "Histology and Immunophenotype of Invasive Lobular Breast Cancer. Daily Practice and Pitfalls." *Breast Dis.* 30: 15–19. doi:10.3233/BD-2009-0278. PMID 19850991.

[8] Rosai Juan,Breast In: Rosai and Ackerman's surgical pathology Volume-2, 10th Ed. *Elsevier;* 2012; 1708-1709.

[9] Orell SR, Sterrett GF, et al; Breat In: Orell and Sterret's Fine Needle Aspiration Cytology, 5th Ed. *Elsevier;* 2012; 193. Bloom HJG, Richardson WW.

[10] Berx G, Cleton-Jansen AM, Strumane K, et al. E-cadherin is inactivated in a majority of invasive human lobular breast cancers by truncation mutations throughout its extracellular domain. *Oncogene* 1996;13:1919-1925.

[11] Nesland JM, Grode TH, Ottestad L, Johannesssen JV. Invasive.lobular carcinoma of the breast. The importance of an alveolar growth pattern. In: Rosen PP, Fechner RE, eds. *Pathology Annual* Vol. 23;1.Norwalk, CT: Appleton & Lange, 1992:233-247.

[12] Fisher ER, Gregorio RM, Redmond C, Fisher B. Tubulolobular invasive breast cancer: a variant of lobular invasive cancer. *Hum Pathol* 1977; 8:679-683.

[13] Dixon JM, Anderson TJ, Page DL, Lee D, Duffy SW. Infiltrating lobular carcinoma of the breast. *Histopathology* 1982;6: 149-161.

[14] Walford N, Ten Velden J. Histiocytoid breast carcinoma: an apocrine variant of lobular carcinoma. *Histopathology* 1989; 14:515-522.

[15] Eusebi V, Magalhaes F, Azzopardi JG. Pleomorphic lobular carcinoma of the breast: an aggressive tumor ~howing apocrine differentiation. *Hum Pathol* 1992;23:655-662.

Chapter 8

Medullary Carcinoma

Medullary carcinoma usually appears in patients under 50 years of age and is said to be particularly common in Japanese women. It is also said to be particularly common in carriers of BRCA1 mutations [1, 2, 3].

Grossly

It is well circumscribed and may become large; it can be mistaken clinically and grossly for a fibroadenoma, but it lacks the trabeculation or whorling of the latter. Its cut surface is solid, homogeneous and gray sometimes exhibiting small foci of necrosis. Rare examples are partially or predominantly cystic [4] (Figure 1).

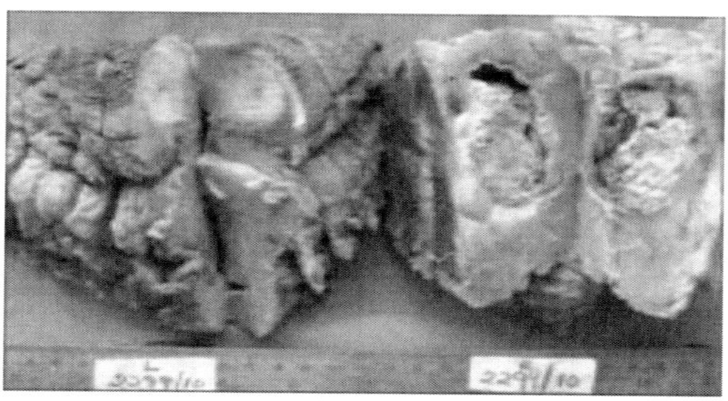

Figure 1. Medullary carcinoma showing well circumscribed and cut surface is solid 'homogenous' and gray.

FNAC (Fine Needle Aspiration Cytology)

It shows highly cellular smear with poorly cohesive cells in clusters and singles. Nuclei are large pleomorphic with prominent nucleoli, many lymphocyte and plasma cells are present [19].

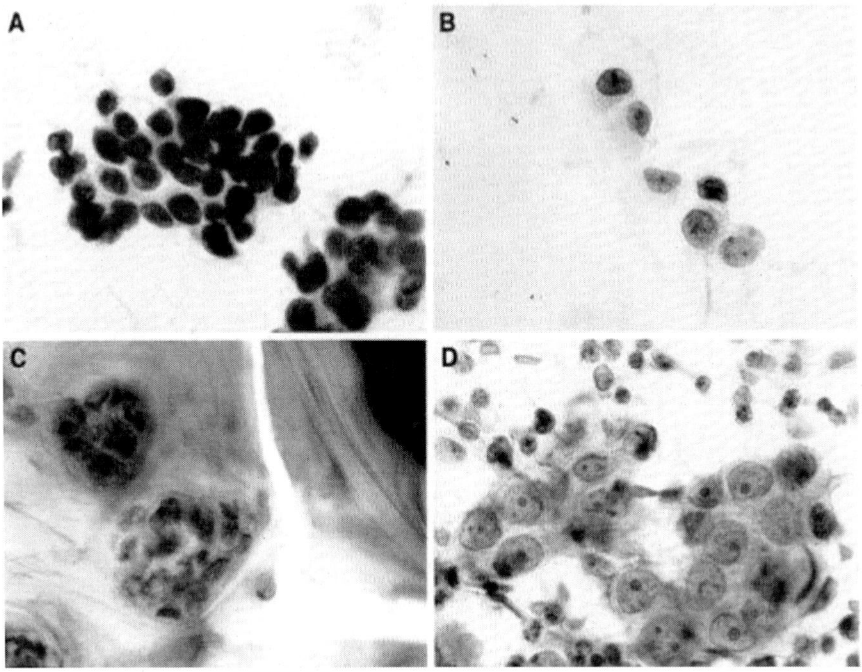

Figure 2. Cytologic features showing medullary carcinoma shows poorly cohesive cell in clusters.

Microscopically

The borders are always of the 'pushing' type. The pattern of growth is diffuse, with minimal or no glandular differentiation or intraductal growth and absence of mucin secretion. The tumor cells are large and pleomorphic, with large nuclei and prominent nucleoli and numerous mitoses (some of them atypical). The cell borders are indistinct, giving the tumor a syncytial or sheet-like appearance somewhat reminiscent of a germ cell tumor of the embryonal carcinoma type. This is accentuated by the fact that the tumor cells located at the periphery of the clusters are more elongated and have a denser, more acidophilic cytoplasm, acquiring a vague resemblance to syncytiotrophoblast. Spindle cell metaplasia, bizarre tumor giant cells, extensive necrosis, and the absence of calcification are other common features. A constant microscopic component is a prominent lymphoplasmacytic infiltrate at the periphery of the tumor, which is thought to represent a reaction of the host tissues to the neoplasm (Figure 20.78) [5, 6, 7, and 8]. The plasma cells are of the IgA-producing type; some of the tumor cells also stain for IgA and for secretory component [9] (Figures 3 and 4).

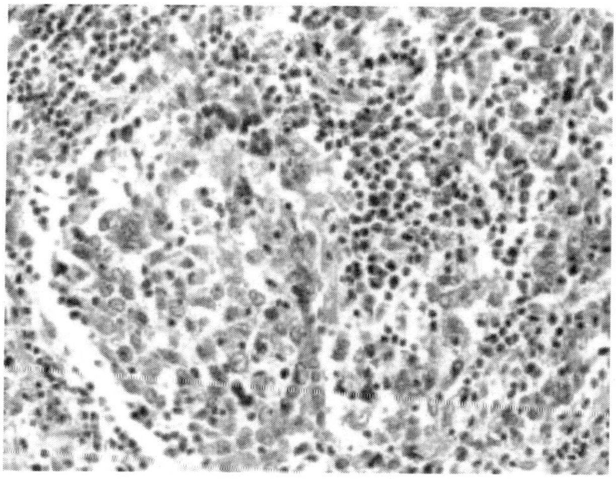

Figure 3. Medullary carcinoma of Breast.

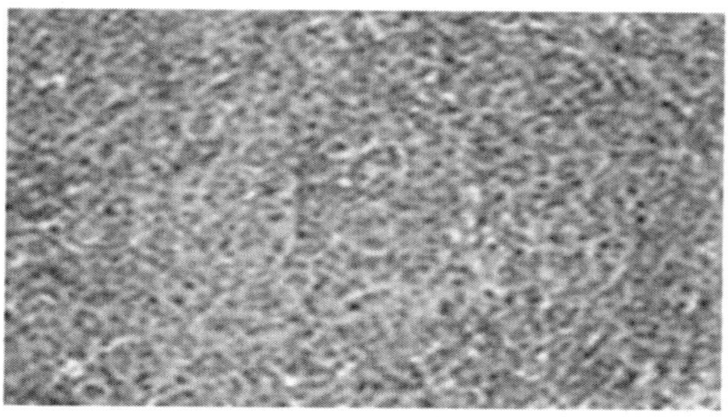

Figure 4. Shows syncytional patteren and lymphoplasmacyticc infiltrate.

Immunohistochemistry

They share the markers of ordinary invasive ductal carcinoma. They typically express CK7, often vimentin, S-100 protein, and P53, but not CK20 [11, 12]. They are almost invariably negative for hormone receptors as well as c-erbB-2 ('triple negative' phenotype) [10]. An interesting feature of medullary carcinoma is the frequent expression of HLA-DR antigen, this being a possible reason for the prominent lymphocytic infiltration [13, 15]. Genetically, medullary carcinoma commonly shows TP53 gene mutation [14] (Figure 5).

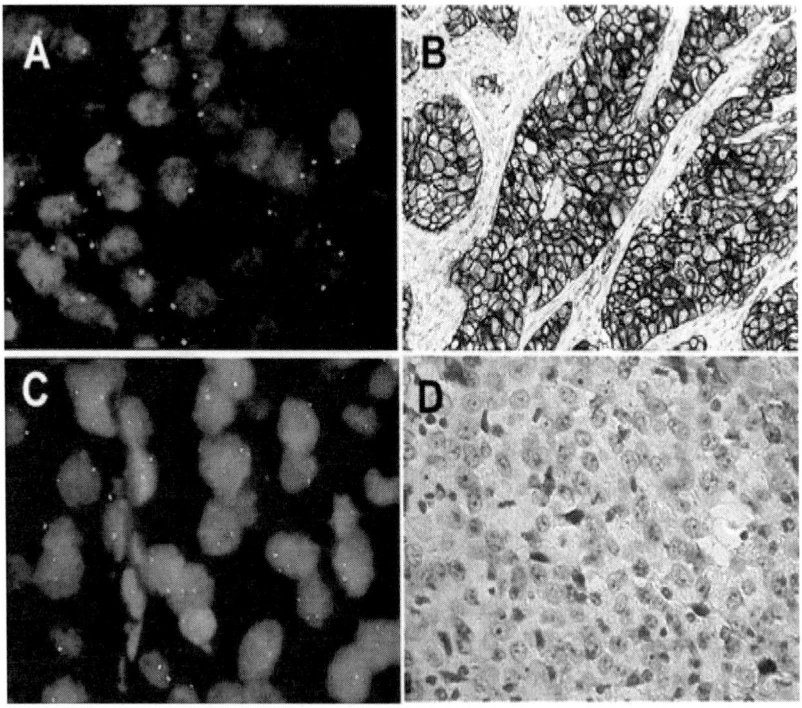

Figure 5. FISH Showing HER 2 Amplification.

Metastasis

Axillary lymph node metastases are common, but they are usually few and limited to the low axillary group.

Prognosis

The prognosis for medullary carcinoma is better than for the ordinary invasive ductal carcinoma, a fact already apparent in the early reports on this tumor [16, 17]. In the series of Ridolfiet al. [18] the 10-year survival rate was 84%, as opposed to 63% for ordinary ductal carcinomas. The prognosis was particularly good for tumors that were smaller than 3 cm, and it remained better than for ductal carcinoma even when nodal metastases were present.

References

[1] Farshid G, Balleine RL, Cummings M, Waring PKathleenCuningham Consortium for Research into Familial Breast Cancer (kConFab): Morphology of breast cancer as a means of triage of patients for BRCA1 genetic testing. *Am J Surg Pathol* 2006; 30:1357-1366.

[2] Armes JE, Venter DJ: The pathology of inherited breast cancer. *Pathology* 2002; 34:309-314.

[3] Shousha S: Medullary carcinoma of the breast and BRCA1 mutation. *Histopathology* 2000; 37:182-185.

[4] Howell LP, Kline TS: Medullary carcinoma of the breast. An unusual cytologic finding in cyst fluid aspirates. *Cancer* 1990; 65:277-282.

[5] Ben-Ezra J, Sheibani K. Antigenic phenotype of the lymphocytic component of medullary carcinoma of the breast. *Cancer* 1987; 59:2037-2041.

[6] Gaffey MJ, Frierson Jr HF, Mills SE, Boyd JC, Zarbo RJ, Simpson JF, Gross LK, Weiss LM: Medullary carcinoma of the breast. Identification of lymphocyte subpopulations and their significance. *Mod Pathol* 1993; 6:721-728.

[7] Kuroda H, Tamaru J, Sakamoto G, Ohnisi K, Itoyama S: Immunophenotype of lymphocytic infiltration in medullary carcinoma of the breast. *Virchows Arch* 2005; 446:10-14.

[8] Yakirevich E, Ben Izhak O, Rennert G, Kovacs ZG, Resnick MB: Cytotoxic phenotype of tumor infiltrating lymphocytes in medullary carcinoma of the breast. *Mod Pathol* 1999; 12:1050-1056.

[9] Hsu S-M, Raine L, Nayak RN: Medullary carcinoma of breast. An immunohistochemical study of its lymphoid stroma. *Cancer* 1981; 48:1368-1376.

[10] Jensen ML, Kiaer H, Andersen J, Jensen V, Melsen F: Prognostic comparison of three classifications for medullary carcinomas of the breast. *Histopathology* 1997; 30:523-532.

[11] Dwarakanath S, Lee AKC, DeLellis RA, Silverman ML, Frasca L, Wolfe HJ: S-100 protein positivity in breast carcinomas. A potential pitfall in diagnostic immunohistochemistry. *Hum Pathol* 1987; 18:1144-1148.

[12] Eichhorn JH: Medullary carcinoma, provocative now as then. *Semin Diagn Pathol* 2004; 21:65-73.

[13] Lazzaro B, Anderson AE, Kajdacsy-Balla A, Hessner MJ: Antigenic characterization of medullary carcinoma of the breast: HLA-DR expression in lymph node positive cases. *Appl Immunohistochem Mol Morphol* 2001; 9:234-241.

[14] Vincent-Salomon A, Gruel N, Lucchesi C, MacGrogan G, Dendale R, Sigal-Zafrani B, Longy M, Raynal V, Pierron G, de Mascarel I, Taris C, Stoppa-Lyonnet D, Pierga JY, Salmon R, Sastre-Garau X, Fourquet A, Delattre O, de Cremoux P, Aurias A: Identification of typical medullary breast carcinoma as a genomic sub-group of basal-like carcinomas, a heterogeneous new molecular entity. *Breast Cancer Res* 2007; 9:R24.

[15] Yazawa T, Kamma H, Ogata T: Frequent expression of HLA-DR antigen in medullary carcinoma of the breast. A possible reason for its prominent lymphocytic infiltration and favorable prognosis. *ApplImmunohistochem* 1993; 1:289-296.

[16] Bloom HJG, Richardson WW, Fields JR: Host resistance and survival in carcinoma of breasts. A study of 104 cases of medullary carcinoma in a series of 1,411 cases of breast cancer followed for 20 years. *Br Med J* 1970; 3:181-188.

[17] Richardson WW: Medullary carcinoma of the breast. A distinctive tumour type with a relatively good prognosis following radical mastectomy. *Br J Cancer* 1956; 10:415-423.

[18] Ridolfi RL, Rosen PP, Port A, Kinne D, Miké V: Medullary carcinoma of the breast. A clinicopathologic study with 10 year follow-up. *Cancer* 1977; 40:1365-1385.

[19] Racz MM, Pommier RF, Troxell ML. Fine needle aspiration cytology of medullary breast carcinoma: Report of 2 cases and review of literature with emphasis on differential diagnosis. D*iagnCytopat*h 2007; 35:313-8.

Chapter 9

Metaplastic Carcinoma

Heterogeneous group of neoplasms with predominant component other than epithelial/glandular.

Terminology

- Also called carcinosarcoma (If mesenchymal component is malignant), carcinoma with osteoclastic giant cells and carcinoma with osseous metaplasia [2, 3].
- "Metaplastic" due to the transformation of epithelial component into a non-glandular component, such as spindle cells, squamous cells or heterologous elements [1].
  - Matrix producing carcinoma: Tumors having overt carcinoma with direct transition to a cartilaginous and/or osseous matrix without an intervening spindle cell zone or osteoclastic giant cell [4, 5].

Clinical Features

- Uncommon (< 5% of breast carcinomas)
- More aggressive than invasive ductal NOS due to larger tumor size, higher grade

- Metastases tend to be hematogenous and not nodal [8, 9, 10)].
- It represents a type of basal-like carcinoma lacking epidermal growth factor receptor and KIT activating mutations, but exhibiting high epidermal growth factor receptor copy number, primarily via aneusomy.

Gross Description

- Well-circumscribed
- Median 3-4 cm, range of size 1-21 cm
- Usually firm, nodular
- Squamous or chondroid areas are pearly white to gray glistening areas on cut surface (Figure 1).

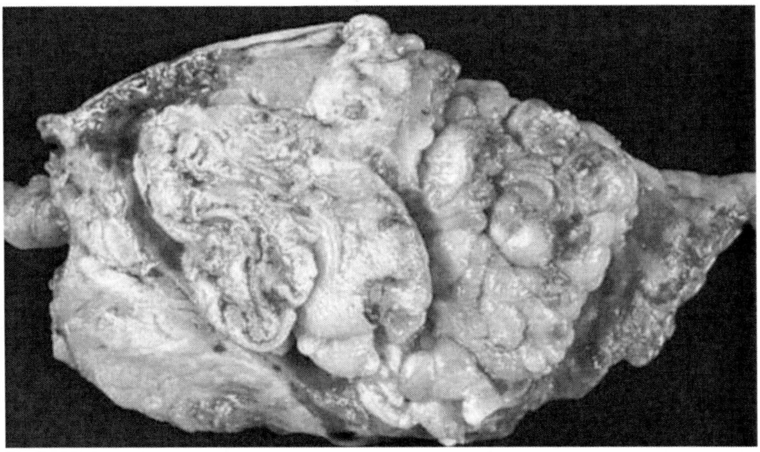

Figure 1. Showing large fleshy mass protruding inside a cavity.

Cytology Description

- Moderate/high cellularity (68%), necrosis (47%), cells are sarcomatoid, poorly differentiated carcinoma or squamous carcinoma
- Dual components usually not identified
- Also clusters of carcinoma cells (Figure 2)

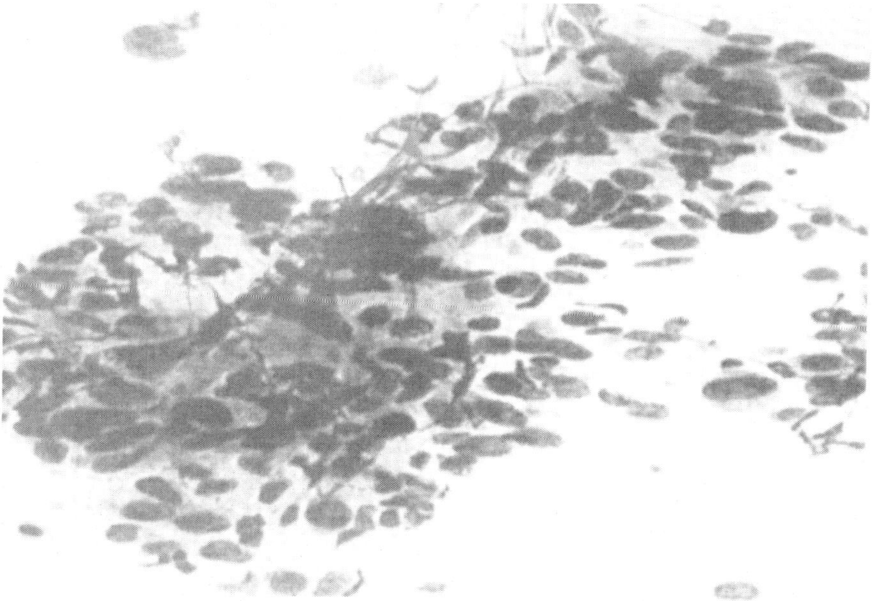

Figure 2. Showing cytological features of Metaplastic carcinoma).

Microscopic Features

- Sarcomatous component resembles fibromatosis (see variant), fibrosarcoma, malignant fibrous histiocytoma, chondrosarcoma or osteosarcoma (see variant), rhabdomyosarcoma, spindle cells (see variant), angiosarcoma or combination
- May need to look carefully for epithelial component (may be ductal carcinoma in situ or invasive ductal carcinoma), may have osteoclast-like giant cells
- Some classify as "with squamous metaplasia" or "with heterologous metaplasia"
- Recommended to test any keratin negative stromal tumor of the breast with myoepithelial markers before calling it a primary sarcoma (Figure 3)

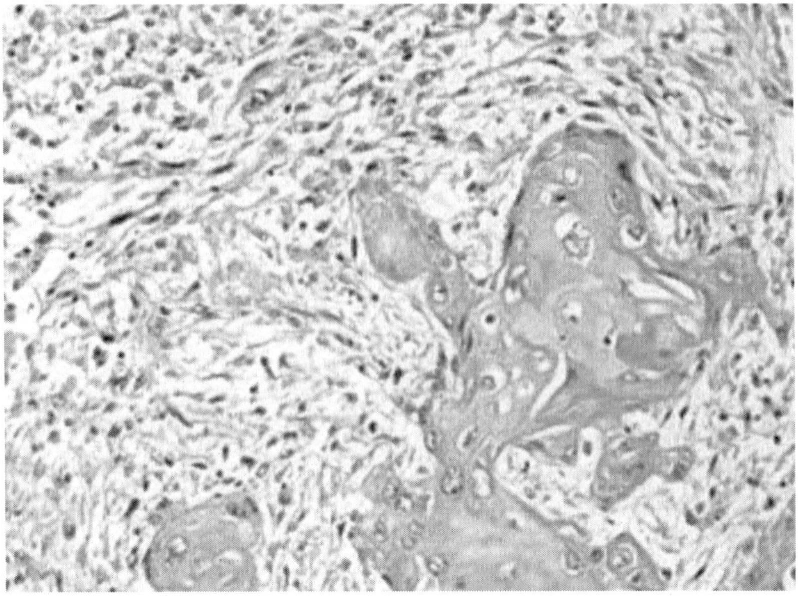

Figure 3. Showing both spindle and squamous component seen.

Immunohistochemistry

- Vimentin in mesenchymal elements
- Keratin (broad spectrum or 34betaE12) in spindle or epithelial cells
- EGFR (76%)
- Squamous components are p63+

Negative stains

- ER, PR, HER2 and mucin
- Often S100
- Mammaglobin [6, 7].

Differential diagnosis

- **Myoepithelial carcinoma:** may have ducts with prominent myoepithelial cells at periphery, diffusely S100+

- **Myofibroblastic tumors**
- **Phyllodes tumor**
- **Primary breast sarcoma:** no epithelial elements or keratin+ elements

References

[1] Harris M, Persaud V: Carcinosarcoma of the breast. *J Pathol* 1974; 112:99-105.

[2] Tavassoli FA: Classification of metaplastic carcinomas of the breast. *Pathol Annu* 1992; 27(Pt 2):89-119.

[3] Wargotz ES, Norris HJ: Metaplastic carcinomas of the breast. III. Carcinosarcoma. *Cancer* 1989; 64:1490-1499.

[4] Downs-Kelly E, Nayeemuddin KM, Albarracin C, Wu Y, Hunt KK, Gilcrease MZ: Matrix-producing carcinoma of the breast: an aggressive subtype of metaplastic carcinoma. *Am J Surg Pathol* 2009; 33:534-541.

[5] Wargotz ES, Norris HJ: Metaplastic carcinomas of the breast. I. Matrix-producing carcinoma. *Hum Pathol* 1989; 20:628-635.

[6] Eusebi V, Cattani MG, Ceccarelli C, Lamovec J: Sarcomatoid carcinomas of the breast. An immunohistochemical study of 14 cases. *Progr Surg Pathol* 1989; 10:83-100.

[7] Santeusanio G, Pascal RR, Bisceglia M, Costantino AM, Bosman C: Metaplastic breast carcinoma with epithelial phenotype of pseudosarcomatous components. *Arch Pathol Lab Med* 1988; 112:82-85.

[8] Carter MR, Hornick JL, Lester S, Fletcher CD: Spindle cell (sarcomatoid) carcinoma of the breast: a clinicopathologic and immunohistochemical analysis of 29 cases. *Am J Surg Pathol* 2006; 30:300-309.

[9] Davis WG, Hennessy B, Babiera G, Hunt K, Valero V, Buchholz TA, Sneige N, Gilcrease MZ: Metaplasticsarcomatoid carcinoma of the breast with absent or minimal overt invasive carcinomatous component: a misnomer. *Am J Surg Pathol* 2005; 29:1456-1463.

[10] Kaufman MW, Marti JR, Gallager HS, Hoehn JL: Carcinoma of the breast with pseudosarcomatous metaplasia. *Cancer* 1984; 53:1908-1917.

Chapetr 10

Adenoid Cystic Carcinoma (ACC) of Breast: An Unusual Breast Malignancy

Introduction

Adenoid cystic carcinomas (ACCs) constitute 0.1–1% of all malignant breast tumors. They have better prognosis than other breast malignancies. To date, there have been about 933 cases reported as per English literature [1, 2]. Adenoid cystic carcinoma (ACC) of the breast is a rare breast cancer variant and optimal management is unclear. Salivary gland tumors having the same histological pattern as ACC of the breast were first termed "cylindroma" by Billroth [3].

Core tip-It is a rare histological diagnosis. Early core biopsy and meticulous histopathological examination is mandatory in each and every palpable breast lump irrespective of age and clinical presentation to prevent untoward complications related to disease and treatment for the sake of accurate pathological diagnosis.

Epidemiology

Although ACC of the breast can occur between 30 and 90 years of age, it is more common in women in the fifth and sixth decade of life, however exceptional cases seen in young age also [4]. Adenoid cystic carcinoma (ACC) of the breast is very rare in males. There have been only eight previous articles published on breast ACC in males [5-13].

Clinical Features

Most patients present with a dominant breast mass tender to palpation [14, 15]. This associated pain has been suggested to be due to the contractile myoepithelial component of these tumours, as perineural invasion is not commonly seen in these lesions [16, 17]. All quadrants seem to be affected, with a particular trend for the peri-areolar region [16].

Diagnostic Evaluation

1) **Fine Needle Aspiration Cytology (FNAC)**The diagnosis can be made on fine needle aspiration cytology [18, 19]. The smears are highly cellular and contain extracellular spheres of metachromatic material surrounded by uniform cells with scant cytoplasm. Cytology reveals atypical epithelial cells with absence of bare nuclei mimicking as atypical epithelial hyperplasia [20] (Figure 1).
2) **The core biopsy** -can be used as an effective diagnostic modality and reveal prominent solid, microcystic, and focally tubuloglandular patterns of growth with intact myoepithelial layer [20] (Figure 2).
3) **Immunohistochemistry**-On immunohistochemical evaluation, the tumor cells are immunopositive for CK7 expression (Figure 3) and myoepithelial cells are positive for p63 (Figure 4).
4) **Histological grading**-The tumor is mostly well circumscribed in appearance and generally ranges from 1 to 5 cm in size [21]. Ro et al. suggested that ACC of the breast can be graded on the proportion of solid growth of the tumor and this was correlated with prognosis [22]. Grades proposed were 1 (no solid element); grade 2 (< 30% solid element); grade 3 (>30% solid element). The proposed treatment was local excision for grade 1 tumors, simple mastectomy for grade 2 tumors and mastectomy with axillary node dissection for grade 3 tumors.

5) **Mammography**-Although calcification may develop in these tumors, only infrequently are they detected by mammography. In one series only 4 of 22 patients detected radiologically [23].
6) **Metastasis**-Axillary lymph node metastases are rare in patients with ACC. Arpino et al. noted lymph node metastases in only 4 of the 182 cases collected from the literature [4]. Distant metastases are uncommon with only 14 cases having been reported, but when they occur they tend to do so without prior lymph node involvement. Hence a routine axillary LN dissection is not recommended [4].
7) **Estrogen Receptor(ER)/progesterone Receptor (PR)** - ACC is generally ER negative; in various series the ER was described as positive in 0.7% to 28% of the cases [23, 24]. PR was positive in 3 of the 13 evaluated patients [23]. Hence; hormonal manipulation is of limited use as most cases are ER & PR negative.

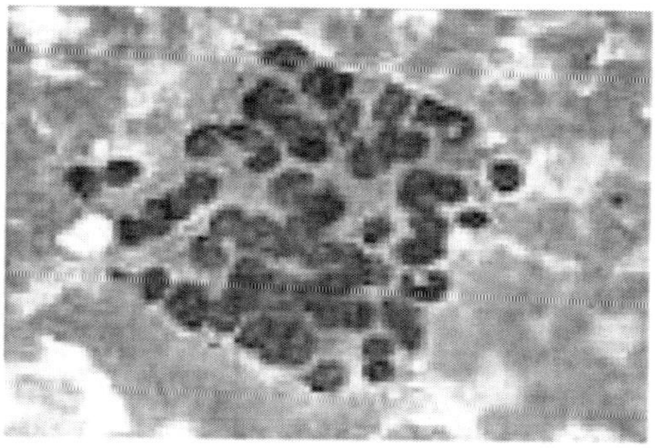

Figure 1. FNAC showing loosely cohesive ductal atypical epithelial cells atypical epithelial hyperplasia.

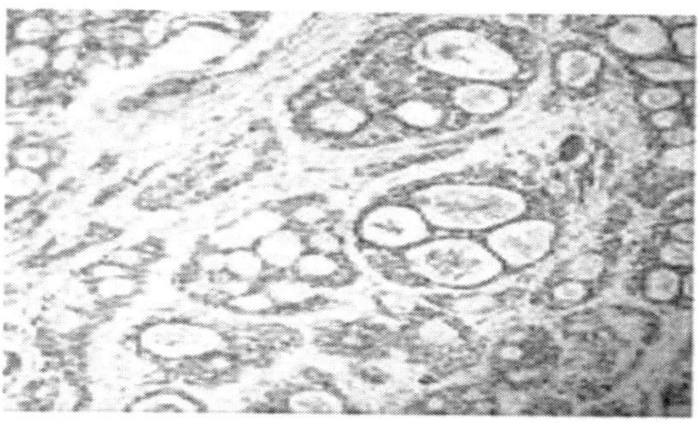

Figure 2. Prominent solid, microcystic, and focally tubuloglandular patterns of growth with intact myoepithelial layer (10×).

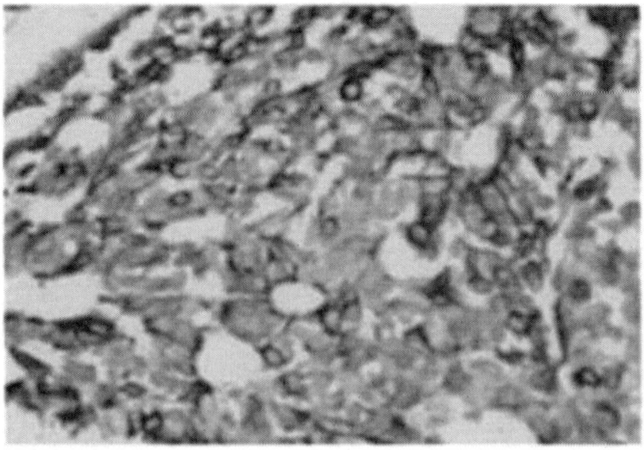

Figure 3. Tumor cells showing cytoplasmic positivity for CK7.

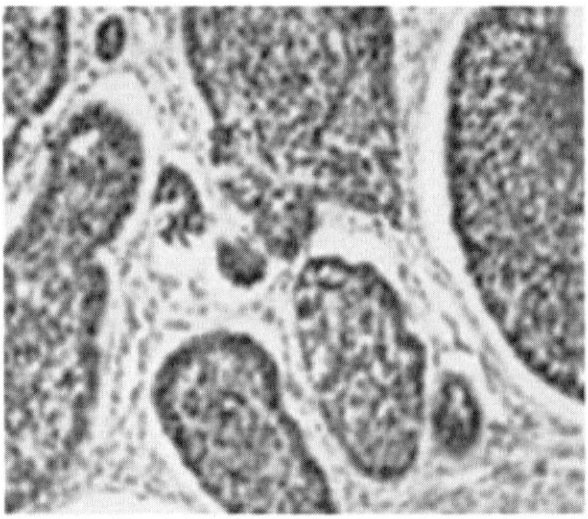

Figure 4. The p63 expression by myoepithelial cells.

Differential Diagnosis

As salivary and mammary glands are exocrine glands both showing a tubulo-acinar architecture, the remarkable similar morphological features observed in tumours arising in these two glandular structures should perhaps not come as a surprise [25]. A good example is offered by salivary duct carcinoma, a lesion that, at the morphological level, is remarkably similar to invasive ductal carcinomas of the breast [26], and that can be categorized in the same molecular subtypes as those identified in invasive ductal breast carcinomas, namely luminal, HER2 and basal subtypes [27].

ACCs constitute an even better example of the similarities between the tumours affecting these sites. ACC of breast and salivary glands share a common pattern of growth, harbour an identical recurrent fusion gene (MYB-NFIB), and similar patterns of numerical chromosomal alterations. Surprisingly, however, despite these similarities, the behaviour of salivary gland and breast ACC differs: while salivary gland lesions have an aggressive behaviour and often metastasise, breast lesions have a much more indolent clinical course.

Treatment and Prognosis

ACC of the breast in females usually has very favorable biological characteristics for treatment [28]. ACC of the breast belongs to the basal-like subgroup of breast cancers [29]. Based on extensive molecular and genetic profiling studies, basal-like tumors are most often hormone receptor (ER and PR) negative and do not express human epidermal growth factor receptor 2 (HER2) [30, 31]. Unlike other triple-negative breast cancers that are associated with poor prognosis, breast ACC has an overall excellent prognosis [28]. The incidents of axillary lymph node metastases and distant metastases are lower [32]. It is because of these distinct clinic-pathologic features that set it apart from the other triple-negative breast cancers [33].

Surgery is a mainstay of treatment for breast ACC. The various options for treatment include lumpectomy, wide excision with or without radical radiation, or modified radical mastectomy. Axillary lymph node dissection is rarely required because of the low incidence of spread to the axillary lymph nodes. Study in ACC of the breast shows that good local control can be achieved by lumpectomy with radiation or by simple mastectomy. Axillary lymph node dissection is worthless considering the rarity of lymph node involvement [4].

Neither adjuvant **chemotherapy nor radiotherapy** guidelines have been studied clearly in patients with ACC of the breast. Although no conclusions have been drawn, the 2011 St. Gallen International Expert Consensus voted that for node-negative breast ACC, adjuvant chemotherapy is not recommended. Radiotherapy is administered when breast-conserving treatment is undertaken, or a large tumor with affected lymph nodes is present [33].

Hormonal treatment and antiHER2 treatment are rarely used, because hormone receptors and HER2/neu expression are usually absent.

Prognosis- Generally, breast ACC has an excellent prognosis compared with other forms of breast cancer and ACC of the salivary glands [34]. Breast ACC does not show the aggressive characteristics of adenoid cystic carcinoma of the salivary gland and has a low local recurrence, a low axillary lymph node involvement, and a rare distant metastasis [33]. The 10-year survival rate for patients with ACC of the breast has ranged from 85% to 100% [28].

References

[1] Alis H, Yigitbas H, Kapan S, Kalayci M, Kilic G, Aygun E. Multifocal adenoid cystic carcinoma of the breast: an unusual presentation. *Can J Surg*. 2008;51(2): E36–E37.

[2] Law YM, Quek ST, Tan PH, Wong SL. Adenoid cystic carcinoma of the breast. *Singapore Med J*. 2009; 50 (1):8–11.

[3] Billroth T: Die Cylindergeschwalst. Untersuchungen ueber die Entwicklung der Blutgefefasse. Berlin: G Reimer; 1856:55-69.

[4] Arpino G, Clark GM, Mohsin S, Bardou VJ, Elledge RM: Adenoid cystic carcinoma of the breast: molecular markers, treatment, and clinical outcome. *Cancer* 94(8):2119-27. Review. 2002 Apr 15.

[5] Kshirsagar AY, Wader JV, Langade YB, Jadhav KP, Zaware SU, Shekhar N. Adenoid cystic carcinoma of the male breast. *Int Surg*. 2006;91:234–6.

[6] Liu J, Jia W, Zeng Y, Deng H, Rao N, Su F. Adolescent male adenoid cystic breast carcinoma. *Am Surg*. 2012;78:E288–9.

[7] Miliauskas JR, Leong AS. Adenoid cystic carcinoma in a juvenile male breast. *Pathology*. 1991;23:298–301.

[8] Yoo SJ, Lee DS, Oh HS, Kim HJ, Kim MH, Ahn YC. Male breast adenoid cystic carcinoma. *Case Rep Oncol*. 2013;6(3):514–9.

[9] Woyke S, Domagala W, Obszewski W. Fine structure of mammary adenoid cystic carcinoma. *Pol Med J*. 1970;9:1140–8.

[10] Verani R, van der Bel-Kahn J. Mammary adenoid cystic carcinoma with unusual features. *Am J Clin Pathol*. 1973;59:653–8.

[11] Ferlito A, Dibonito L. Adenoid cystic carcinoma of the male breast, report of a case. *Am Surg*. 1974;40:72–6.

[12] Hjorth S, Magnusson PH, Blomquist P. Adenoid cystic carcinoma of the breast. *Acta Chir Scand*. 1977;143:155–8.

[13] Tang et al. Breast adenoid cystic carcinoma in a 19-year-old man: a case report and review of the literature. *World Journal of Surgical Oncology* (2015) 13:19 DOI 10.1186/s12957-015-0442-8.

[14] Anthony PP, James PD: Adenoid cystic carcinoma of the breast: prevalence, diagnostic criteria, and histogenesis. *J Clin Pathol* 1975, 28(8):647-55.

[15] Lusted D: Structural and growth patterns of adenoid cystic carcinoma of breast. *Am J clin Pathol* 1970, 54(3):419-25.

[16] Rosen PP. Adenoid cystic carcinoma. In: Rosen PP, ed. Rosen's breast pathology. Philadelphia: Lippincott Williams and Wilkins, 2009:590e604.

[17] Bennett AK, Mills SE, Wick MR. Salivary-type neoplasms of the breast and lung. *Semin Diagn Pathol* 2003;20:279-304.

[18] Culubret M, Roig I: Fine needle aspiration biopsy of adenoid cystic carcinoma of the breast: a case report. *Diagn Cytopathol* 1996, 15(5):431-4.

[19] Stanley MW, Tani EM, Rutquist LE, Skoog L: Adenoid cystic carcinoma of the breast: diagnosis by fine needle aspiration. *Diagn Cytopathol* 1993, 9(2):184-7.

[20] Sachin B. Ingle, Nawab P. Jamadar, Baban D. Adgaonkar, Chitra R. Hinge (Ingle) and Saleha Siddiqui. An Interesting Pathological Diagnosis – Adenoid Cystic Carcinoma in an Adolescent Girl. *Breast Cancer: Basicand Clinical Research* 2015:9.

[21] Cavanzo FJ, Taylor HB: Adenoid cystic carcinoma of the breast. *An analysis of 21 cases. Cancer* 1969, 24(4):740-5.

[22] Ro JY, Silva EG, Gallager HS: Adenoid cystic carcinoma of the breast. *Hum Pathol* 1987, 18(12):1276-81. Review.

[23] McClenathan JH, de la Roza G: Adenoid cystic breast cancer. *Am J Surg* 2002, 183(6):646-9.

[24] Leeming R, Jenkins M, Mendelsohn G: Adenoid cystic carcinoma of the breast. *Arch Surg* 1992, 127(2):233-5. Review.

[25] Foschini MP, Reis-Filho JS, Eusebi V, et al. Salivary gland-like tumours of the breast: surgical and molecular pathology. *J Clin Pathol* 2003;56:497e506.

[26] Perou CM, Sorlie T, Eisen MB, et al. Molecular portraits of human breast tumours. *Nature* 2000;406:747e52.

[27] Di Palma S, Skalova A, Ungari M, et al. Pure salivary duct carcinomas can be classified into luminal, Her2 and basal-like phenotypes. Abstract 1072. *Mod Pathol* 2008;21(Suppl 1).

[28] Boujelbene N, Khabir A, Boujelbene N, Jeanneret Sozzi W, Mirimanoff RO, Khanfir K. Clinical review- breast adenoid cystic carcinoma. *Breast*.2012;21:124–7.

[29] Sorlie T, Tibshirani R, Parker J, Hastie T, Marron JS, Nobel A, et al. Repeated observation of breast tumor subtypes in independent gene expression data sets. *Proc Natl Acad Sci U S A*. 2003;100:8418–23.

[30] Miyai K, Schwartz MR, Divatia MK, Anton RC, Yong Wook P, Ayala AG, et al. Adenoid cystic carcinoma of breast: recent advances. *World J Clin Cases*. 2014;2(12):732–41.

[31] Rakha EA, Elsheikh SE, Aleskandarany MA, Habashi HO, Green AR, Powe DG, et al. Triple-negative breast cancer: distinguishing between basal and nonbasal subtypes. *Clin Cancer Res*. 2009;15:2302–10.

[32] Peters GN, Wolff M. Adenoid cystic carcinoma of the breast. Report of 11 new cases: review of the literature and discussion of biological behaviour. *Cancer*. 1983;52:680–6.

[33] Ghabach B, Anderson WF, Curtis RE, Huycke MM, Lavigne JA, Dores GM. Adenoid cystic carcinoma of the breast in the United States (1977–2006): a population-based cohort study. *Breast Cancer Res*. 2010; 12(4):R54.

[34] Li N, Xu L, Zhao H, El-Naggar AK, Sturgis EM. A comparison of the demographics, clinical features, and survival of patients with adenoid cystic carcinoma of major and minor salivary glands versus less common sites within the Surveillance, Epidemiology, and End Results registry. *Cancer*. 2012;118:3945–53.

Chapter 11

Papillary Carcinoma of Breast

Introduction

Papillary carcinoma (PC) of the breast, which accounts for 0.5% to 1% of breast cancer, is a distinct histological subtype that is characterized by malignant epithelial proliferation supported by fibrovascular stalks [1-10]. PC can be either localized, forming an expansile mass corresponding to intracystic/encysted (IPC) and solid (SPC) variants of PC, or it can diffuse within terminal duct lobular units and correspond to papillary variant of ductal carcinoma in situ (papillary DCIS) [3, 8, 10-13]. Compared with IPC, SPC is typically solid, characterized by mucin production and neuroendocrine features, and is more often multinodular [13, 14], whereas papillary DCIS is typically surrounded by a peripheral layer of myoepithelial cells [3, 11]. These lesions usually present as subareolar mass and/or nipple discharge [11]. The term encapsulated PC (EPC) has recently been introduced to define IPC [15-17] and SPC [13, 14] that are typically circumscribed and often encapsulated (separated from the surrounding mammary stroma by a fibrous capsule) and lack myoepithelial cells at their periphery.

Epidemiology

1) Age- The intracystic papillary carcinoma is more frequently found among postmenopausal women with an average age between 55 and 67 years old.

2) Sex Predilection-IPC is extremely rare in males [18-20]. The clinical presentation in males is similar to that in females except for a higher median age in males (60 vs. 53 years) [19].
3) Incidence- An analysis of the California Cancer Registry provides a more specific analysis of intracystic papillary carcinoma. Between 1988 and 2005, a total of 917 cases were identified from this population-based registry. Of these, 427 were classified as intracystic papillary carcinoma *in situ*, whereas 490 cases were classified as invasive disease. The median age reported in this series was 69.5 years (range 27 to 99 years), with 3.5% of diagnoses occurring in men. Notably, the male incidence of intracystic papillary carcinoma appears to be substantially higher than the total reported incidence of male breast cancer (constituting approximately 1% of invasive tumors). Looking specifically at cases of invasive cancers, the majority of cases were localized at the time of diagnosis (89.6%). Approximately 7.8% of cases were noted to have associated regional disease, with extension into adjacent tissue or axillary involvement, and only 2 cases (0.4%) possessed distant metastases at the time of diagnosis [20, 21].

Pathophysiology

The causative risk factors include age, genetics, family history, diet, alcohol, Obesity, lifestyle, physical inactivity, as well as endocrine factors (both endogenous and exogenous). Other associated factors for breast cancer are mammographic density and previous benign disease. However, it is still not very clear which of the factors has any predominant role over others, in the pathogenesis of breast cancer.

Age

Russell [22] observed that breast cancer is very uncommon before twenty years of age, but the incidence gradually increases with age, and by the age of ninety years, one fifth of women are affected. In addition to that, Dumitrescu and Cotarla [23] reported that less than 10 new cases were recorded per 100,000 women below 25 years, and increased up to 100 times by the age of

45 years. This indicates that the reproductive hormones produced by the ovaries and the adrenal glands are involved in the pathogenesis of breast cancer, since cancers that are not responsive to hormones will not show any appreciable change of incidence during the female reproductive period [24].

Furthermore, it is also believed that the age at menarche and menopause contribute to the duration of exposure to the carcinogenic effects of the gonadal (sex) hormones. In support of this Aguas et al. [25] observed that the risk of breast cancer reduces 15-20% for each year that menarche is delayed, and that late menopause at 55 years or older is a risk factor. This is because early menarche and delayed menopause will increase the duration of estrogen exposure during a woman's reproductive years, but there has to be collaboration with genetic and Environmental factors for breast cancer to develop.

Gender

Only less than one percent of patients with breast cancer are males [22]. However, the differences are thought to be hormonal since even the male breast cancer has been shown to express oestrogen, progesterone and androgen receptors and men with Klinefelter's syndrome have been observed to have increased chance of developing breast cancer [26].

Genetic Factors

Breast cancer is more common in women with a family history compared to the general population. Russell [22] observed that only about 5% of breast cancers are related to a specific mutation. Also, a meta-analysis of 52 separate epidemiological studies revealed that 12% of women with this disease have one affected family member and 1% of the patients have one or more relatives affected. The study concluded that women with one or more first degree relatives affected with breast cancer have higher breast cancer risk than those who don't [23].

Diet and Alcohol

Diet and Alcohol are thought to play a role in the etiology of breast cancer, and there is a link between diets low in phyto-oestrogens and this disease, as well as high intake of alcohol [22]. According to Dumitrescu and Cotarla [23] the risk increases progressively in a dose-dependent manner to an alcohol intake of 60 g (2-5 drinks) per day, depending on the strength of the drink, and for every 10 g increment (approximately 0.75-1 L drink) in daily alcohol consumption, the risk increases with 9%.

Furthermore, well-cooked meat and diets rich in fats are associated with increased incidence of breast cancer, and it has been observed that diets containing 35-40% of fat in calories like most Western diets have a mammary tumor-producing effect [25]. This is because high fat diets are rich in cholesterol which is a precursor in the synthesis of oestrogens and other steroid hormones, therefore exposing the breast to higher amounts of estrogen which can stimulate the development of cancer. It was also observed that dietary fiber ingestion inhibits the Intestinal resorption of estrogens and this protection is higher with a daily intake of 35-45 g of dietary fiber [25].

Obesity Lifestyle and Physical Activity

Along with diet, exercise can interfere with plasma levels of hormones which may influence breast cancer development. Aguas et al. [25] observed that these two factors separately or in combination influence the body weight and obesity increases the risk of breast cancer in post-menopausal women. Dumitrescu and Cotarla [23] supported this observation in their paper and noted that breast cancer risk is particularly evident among obese women who don't use hormone replacement therapy, and for each 5 kg of weight gain, breast cancer risk increases by 8%. This is explained by the fact that fat in adipose tissue is an important source of estrogens, which are synthesized from cholesterol.

Endocrine Factors (Endogenous)

Breast cancer is more commonly seen in infertile women and those who don't breast-feed their babies. First full-term pregnancy at an early age, especially if associated with late menarche and early menopause (which decrease the duration of oestrogen exposure of a woman) has been found to be protective [22]. Both early age (less than 20 years versus 30 years) at first full-term pregnancy and higher parity decrease breast cancer risk to half of the risk of women that didn't bear children. This is because the level of estrogen is lower in pregnancy and in women that had many children [23].

Exogenous Factors

A large meta-analysis demonstrated that long-term hormone replacement therapy (HRT) is responsible for the cumulative excess of breast tumors over those expected in women between 50-70 years [23]. Aguas et al. [25] also reported that hormone replacement therapy (HRT) is associated with an increased risk of breast cancer (with a relative risk of 1.21-1.40), especially among current users of estrogen plus progestin for five years and longer.

The same is true for oral contraceptives as the report showed a modest increase in breast cancer risk associated with current and recent use, with a relative risk of 1.24 reported in a meta-analysis of 54 studies involving 150,000 women. The risk is believed to be greater for those who began contraception before 20 years of age [25]. Dumitrescu et al. [23] also demonstrated a connection between breast cancer and oral contraceptive use independent of dose, age of first use, length of use, age of diagnosis or a family history of breast cancer. The risk is attributed to the estrogen content of the contraceptives, which contributes to the Pathogenesis of breast cancer. Again, it is important to point out the obvious advantages of oral contraceptives in preventing unwanted and untimely pregnancies, as well as giving individuals choice in planning their families.

Molecular Genetics of Breast Cancer

Five to ten percent of all breast cancers arise from germ-line mutations in high-penetrance breast cancer susceptibility genes such as BRCA1, BRCA2, p53 and PTEN, and confer a high individual risk for developing hereditary breast cancer [23]. The BRCA1 gene is located on the long arm of chromosome 17, while BRCA2 is located on the long arm of chromosome 13. Gene-positive patients have an 80% risk of developing breast cancer especially in the pre-menopausal age group [22]. Aguas et al. [25] observed that BRCA1 and BRCA2 predispose a woman to breast cancer in only 5-10% of the total number of breast cancers and believe that even though family history may reflect shared genes, it may also suggest shared environmental lifestyle exposures. They therefore advised that due to ethical and legal issues, as well

[26] as psychological consequences, genetic screening should only be carried out in the research settings, rather than in routine clinical practice. But we know that genetic screening is carried out selectively in affectedfamilies.

The Role of HER-2/neu Antigen

HER-2/neu Antigen is a growth factor protein which is over-expressed in different types of human cancers, including breast, ovarian, lung, gastric, and oral cancers [27]. In 1987, the HER-2/neu proto-oncogene was revealed to be amplified and over-expressed in 20-30% of invasive breast cancers, and also shown to be associated with poorer outcome and shortened survival [28]. In addition, HER-2/neu-positivity is thought to predict the likelihood of resistance or sensitivity to some conventional hormonal therapies like Tamoxifen. Herceptin (Trastuzumab), a recombinant humanized anti-HER-2/neu monoclonal antibody has been shown to improve outcomes for women with metastatic breast cancer, either alone or in combination with chemotherapy [29].

Steroid Hormones and Their Receptors

It has also been observed that breast stromal cells can modulate the growth of normal and neoplastic breast epithelial cells and can secrete growth factors following stimulation by endogenous hormones. The adipose tissues contain aromatase enzyme which produces oestradiol from circulating cholesterol. Because of the higher proportion of these fat cells in breasts of older women, the levels of oestradiol in breast tissues of post-menopausal women are much greater than their plasma levels [30]. This probably accounts for the rising incidence of breast cancer with ageing and supports the role of steroid hormones in the pathogenesis of breast cancer.

Steroid hormone receptors are structurally-related intra-cellular proteins that bind to steroid hormones such as oestrogens and progesterone and relay their signals leading to down-stream gene expression (signal transduction). Cancers dependent on steroid hormones include breast, prostate, testicular, ovarian and endometrial cancer which result from deregulation of hormone secretion, signaling and receptor action [24]. The concept of steroid hormone playing an important role in carcinogenesis was first demonstrated by surgical removal of the ovaries, which was followed by reduced levels of circulating hormones and remarkable improvement in women with breast cancer [31]. Estrogen is now believed to mediate its various functions through two specific intra-cellular receptors estrogen receptor- α and β (ER-α and ER-β), which are produced by different genes and function as ligand-activated transcription factors [32]. These, along with androgen receptors (AR) are the members of the nuclear hormone receptor superfamily which form homo-dimers and bind specific DNA elements called Hormone responsive elements (HRE) in the target gene promoters [33].

Clinical Presentation

Intracystic papillary breast cancer usually occurs in elderly postmenopausal women. This form of breast cancer has a very subtle clinical presentation of a painless breast lump which could be present for a long duration or bloody nipple discharge. There are only a few cases reported in the literature of IPC occurring in younger women of less than 40 years old [34, 35].

Diagnostic Evaluation

Carter et al. classified breast papillary lesions into invasive and non-invasive papillary carcinoma with the latter being sub-divided into two types [12]. The first one is a diffuse form, the papillary variant of DCIS, which includes medium and small ducts, and the second one is a localized form, intracystic (encysted) papillary carcinoma, which is a solitary tumour in a cystic and dilated duct. There are three main subtypes of intracystic papillary breast cancer (IPC), IPC alone (pure form), IPC with surrounding DCIS, and IPC with invasion [34].

Mammography

Radiological findings may show on a mammography as a round, oval or lobulated opacity. The margins of the mass are usually circumscribed, but may be obscured or indistinct at places testifying inflammation or invasion. The differential diagnosis on mammography in the age group of these tumors includes hematoma, invasive ductal carcinoma, colloid or medullary carcinoma, benign cyst or adenofibroma [35].

Sonography

At sonography, intracystic papillary carcinoma appears as single or predominantly cystic masses, with or without septa and with solid papillary mass projecting into the cystic lumen from the inner wall demonstrating vascular flow within the solid component of the cystic mass on a color Doppler scan [36, 45]. Although some radiologic features, such as posterior acoustic enhancement and associated microcalcifications, are more frequently associated with malignancy, the radiologic appearance cannot accurately predict the behaviour of papillary lesions, and histologic evaluation is necessary [43].

Magnetic Resonance Imaging

Magnetic resonance imaging of the breast with contrast enhancement can further aid in the diagnosis showing enhanced cyst wall, septation, and mural nodules [37].

Cytology

Cytological diagnosis may be misleading as you can aspirate the fluid within the cystic component of the lesion which could be negative for malignancy and therefore give a false negative result. Fine Needle Aspiration Cytology confirms the presence of atypical cells [1] (Figure 1). Vacuum-assisted ultrasound-guided core biopsy would be superior to FNAC in suspected cases [38]. A core biopsy of the lesion reveals atypical ductal hyperplasia, but no evidence of malignancy [1]. The core biopsy targets the central part of the solid tumour, while the invasion usually occurs at the periphery; therefore, excision biopsy of B3 papillary lesions is recommended to exclude invasive cancer or associated adjacent DCIS [38]. Tomonori et al. [10], also suggested necessity of excisional biopsy. Visualizing the intraductal papillary lesions by mammary ductoscopy has been described to be a valuable tool in diagnosing such lesions [39]. However, the potential of this technique in management of IPC requires further investigation.

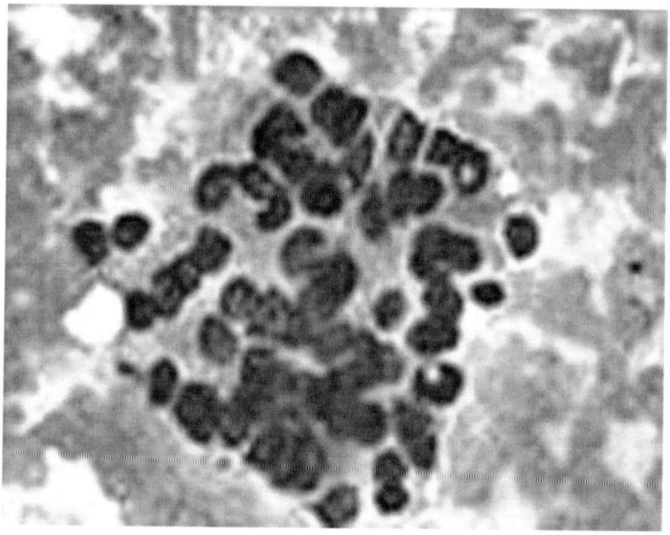

Figure 1. Fine Needle Aspiration Cytology confirmed the presence of atypical cells.

Histology

Intracystic papillary carcinoma is accepted as a borderline lesion in progression from insitu to invasive carcinoma because histologically there is scanty or no MEC layer a situation similar to invasive carcinoma [40-42]. Histology of insitu intracystic papillary tumor shows papillary, adenoid and cribriform structures lined by columnar cells exhibiting features of marked cytological atypia, i.e., nuclear hyperchromasia, pleomorphism, abnormal mitosis and increased N:C ratio (Nucleocytoplasmic ratio) with fibro vascular cores [1] (Figure 2). It is histologically characterized by one or several nodules of papillary carcinoma surrounded by a fibrous capsule, it may have various cellular patterns (cribriform, stratified spindle cell, compact columnar epithelial or transitional cell form) or a combination of patterns and shows typical histological findings, which are low or intermediate nuclear grade, absence of necrosis [43]. High nuclear grade and the presence of necrosis seem to be indicator of more aggressive tumors [44].

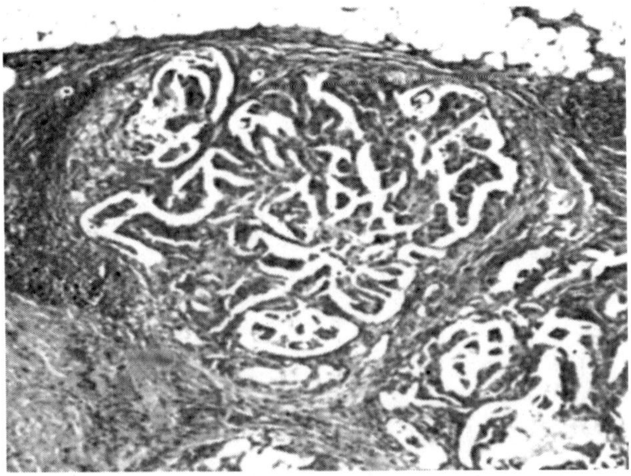

Figure 2. Showing intraductalmalignant cells arranged in papillary fronds exhibiting features of malignancy (Insitu Papillary Carcinoma of Breast), × 10.

A minority of encapsulated papillary carcinomas may be associated with a component of invasive carcinoma. The invasive component is characterized by an infiltrative appearance with extension beyond the fibrous capsule of the lesion. Invasive areas in general do not display papillary features but rather exhibit the morphology of an invasive ductal carcinoma not otherwise specified [43].

Fine needle aspiration and core needle biopsy may be unable to differentiate between insitu and invasive lesions as invasion is often identified at the periphery of the tumor. Therefore surgical excision is performed for adequate histologic diagnosis and treatment [44, 45].

Differential Diagnosis

Invasive features into the stroma, higher nuclear grade & necrosis differentiates the IPC from the Intracystic (encapsulated) papillary breast (EPC) which is usually of low or intermediate nuclear grade with no evidence of necrosis, strongly ER receptor positive, negative for C-erb2(Her2neu) [46].

Differential diagnoses also include benign & malignant lesions like atypical ductal hyperplasia (ADH), lobular hyperplasia & DCIS. Fibrovascular cores are absent in ADH & the cellular discohesion is the pathognomic feature of lobular neoplasms [47].

DCIS do not show branching fibrovascular stroma but IPC can show DCIS component along with IDC exhibiting pure mucinous, neuroendocrine or rarely lobular or tubular carcinoma [47]. Gruber et al. in his study of radiological breast cancer evaluation using various modalities concluded that Magnetic resonance imaging (MRI) & Mammogram are more exact cancer sizing techniques whilst USG showed significant underestimation [48].

Immunohistochemistry (IHC) has an important role in hormonal, invasion assessment. Papillary carcinomas of the breast tend to be ER, PR receptors positive & Her2Neu negative [47, 49, 50]. IHC markers for MCL have an important role in invasion assessment with smooth muscle actin, p63, CD10, S-100, calponin, maspin commonly employed among which smooth muscle myosin heavy chain & p63 are more MCL specific [50, 51].

Treatment

Variable management strategies are considered when dealing with this rare form of breast cancer. Treatment options for the breast can involve breast conserving surgery in the form of wide local excision, with or without adjuvant RT, or mastectomy [9]. Axillary interventions,including sentinel lymph node biopsy (SLNB), and/or axillary dissection (AD) [52] and adjuvant systemic treatment which have mainly involved endocrine manipulation with Tamoxifen as this cancer seems to be almost certainly hormonal positive and HER-2 negative [53]. Despite these general principles, the optimal management of IPC remains controversial.

The low yield for metastasis and vascular invasion make chemotherapeutic intervention not mandatory. This treatment modality would be only considered in cases associated with lymphovascular invasion and can be safely omitted in IPC alone or with associated DCIS. Furthermore, the balance of benefit and risk has been influenced by the good clinical prognosis which is reported in such cases [54].

Surgery

Irrespective of the type of surgery, the rate of recurrence and the probabilities of dying from IPC do not differ between the three groups [9]. In the cases of IPC alone, IPC with DCIS, or IPC with invasion, complete local excision of the tumour with clear margins is the recommended surgical treatment [55]. However, radical or modified radical mastectomy is not indicated for the treatment of pure IPC as this is a low-grade form of cancer, especially in elderly women in whom it so often occurs. Nevertheless, in some cases skin-sparing mastectomy with or without immediate breast reconstruction can be offered (e.g., large tumours, inadequate margins, recurrence, and patient preference). Axillary lymph node surgery in the form of SLNB is considered prudent in IPC; as it rarely metastasizes, in order to spare patients from the morbidity of axillary node clearance in node negative cases.

Radiotherapy

Research to support the theory that adjuvant radiotherapy significantly reduces the risk of LR in those undergoing breast conserving surgery in cases of IPC is still ongoing. However, many articles and published data recommend adjuvant RT for IPC associated with invasion and or DCIS [53]. Moreover, in young women (less than 50 years), with IPC alone, radiotherapy has been suggested as an adjuvant treatment [9, 53].

Oncological Therapy

Systemic adjuvant therapy has focused on endocrine manipulation, principally the use of Tamoxafin as IPC tends to be ER/PR Positive and HER 2 negative, although there is no clear indication for adjuvant endocrine therapy. Given that the overall good prognosis and that there is no adjuvant treatment which increases cancer-free survival, there is a concern for potential overtreatment in this disease [16]. Nonetheless, in young (less than 50 years old) patients with pure IPC and associated DCIS or micro-invasion, there is some evidence to suggest that adjuvant radiation and endocrine therapy should be considered to reduce the risk of local recurrence [53].

References

[1] Sachin B Ingle, Chitra R Hinge (Ingle), Hemant G Murdeshwar, Baban D Adgaonkar. Unusual case of insitu (intracystic) papillary carcinoma of Breast. *World J Clin Cases* 2013 October 16; 1(7): 227-229.

[2] Anderson WF, Chu KC, Chang S, et al. Comparison of age-specific incidence rate patterns for different histopathologic types of breast carcinoma. *Cancer Epidemiol Biomarkers Prev*. 2004;13:1128–1135.

[3] Collins LC, Schnitt SJ. Papillary lesions of the breast: selected diagnostic and management issues. Histopathology. 2008;52:20–29.

[4] Fayanju OM, Ritter J, Gillanders WE, et al. Therapeutic management of intracystic papillary carcinoma of the breast: the roles of radiation and endocrine therapy. *Am J Surg*. 2007;194:497–500.

[5] Koerner F. Papilloma and papillary carcinoma. *Semin Diagn Pathol*. 2010;27:13–30.

[6] Li CI, Uribe DJ, Daling JR. Clinical characteristics of different histologic types of breast cancer. *Br J Cancer*. 2005;93:1046–1052.

[7] Louwman MW, Vriezen M, van Beek MW, et al. Uncommon breast tumors in perspective: incidence, treatment and survival in the Netherlands. *Int J Cancer*. 2007;121:127–135.

[8] Pal SK, Lau SK, Kruper L, et al. Papillary carcinoma of the breast: an overview. *Breast Cancer Res Treat*. 2010;122:637–645.

[9] Solorzano CC, Middleton LP, Hunt KK, et al. Treatment and outcome of patients with intracystic papillary carcinoma of the breast. *Am J Surg*. 2002;184:364–368.

[10] Ueng SH, Mezzetti T, Tavassoli FA. Papillary neoplasms of the breast: a review. *Arch Pathol Lab Med*. 2009;133:893–907.

[11] MacGrogan G, Moinfar F, Raju U. Pathology and genetics of tumors of the breast and female genital organs. In: Tavassoli FA Devilee P. World Health Organization Classification of Tumors. Lyon: *IACR Press*; 2003.

[12] Carter D, Orr SL, Merino MJ. Intracystic papillary carcinoma of the breast: after mastectomy, radiotherapy or excisional biopsy alone. *Cancer*. 1983;52:14–19.

[13] Rosen PP. Rosen's Breast Pathology. Philadelphia: Lippincott Williams & Wilkins; 2009:423–449.

[14] Wei B, Bu H, Chen HJ, et al. Clinicopathologic study of solid papillary carcinoma of breast. *Zhonghua Bing Li Xue Za Zhi*. 2006;35:589–593.

[15] Calderaro J, Espie M, Duclos J, et al. Breast intracystic papillary carcinoma: an update. *Breast J*. 2009;15:639–644.

[16] Collins LC, Carlo VP, Hwang H, et al. Intracystic papillary carcinomas of the breast: a reevaluation using a panel of myoepithelial cell markers. *Am J Surg Pathol*. 2006;30:1002–1007.

[17] Hill CB, Yeh IT. Myoepithelial cell staining patterns of papillary breast lesions: from intraductal papillomas to invasive papillary carcinomas. *Am J Clin Pathol.* 2005;123:36–44.

[18] Laszio R, O'Brian ME, Relihan N, et al. Intracystic papillary carcinoma in a male as a rare presentation of breast cancer: A case report and literature review. *J Med Case Reports* 2009;3: 13.

[19] Arora R, Gupta R, Sharma A, et al. Invasive papillary carcinoma of male breast. *Ind J Pathol Microbiol* 2010;53: 135-37.

[20] Dragoumis DM, Tsiftsoglou AP. Intracystic papillary carcinoma associated with ductal carcinoma in-situ in male breast. *Images in Pathology* 2008;54: 39-40.

[21] Grabowski J, Salzstein SL, Sadler GR, Blair S. Intracystic papillary carcinoma. *Cancer.* 2008;113(5):916–20.

[22] Russell (2000) Bailey and Love's Short Practice of Surgery. In Chapter on breast cancer (23rdedn) Arnold, London.

[23] Dumitrescu RG, Cotarla I (2005) Understanding breast cancer risk -- where do we stand in 2005? *J Cell Mol Med* 9: 208-221.

[24] Sabiston DC, Lyerly HK (1997) Sabiston textbook of surgery: The biological basis of modern surgical practice (fifteenth edn) Philadelphia, Pennsylvania: WB Saunders Company.

[25] Aguas F, Martins A, Gomes TP, de Sousa M, Silva DP; Portuguese Menopause Society and Portuguese Gynaecology Society (2005) Prophylaxis approach to a-symptomatic post-menopausal women: *breast cancer. Maturitas* 52: S23-31.

[26] Murphy CE, Carder PJ, Lansdown MR, Speirs V (2006) Steroid hormone receptor expression in male breast cancer. *Eur J Surg Oncol* 32: 44-47.

[27] Hung MC, Lau YK (1999) Basic science of HER-2/neu: a review. *Semin Oncol* 26: 51-59.

[28] Gancberg D, Lespagnard L, Rouas G, Paesmans M, Piccart M, et al. (2000) Sensitivity of HER-2/neu antibodies in archival tissue samples of invasive breast carcinomas. Correlation with oncogene amplification in 160 cases. *Am J Clin Pathol* 113: 675-682.

[29] Baselga J, Tripathy D, Mendelsohn J, Baughman S, Benz CC, et al. (1999) Phase II study of weekly intravenous Trastuzumab (Herceptin) in patients with HER-2/neu-overexpressing metastatic breast cancers. *Seminars in oncology* 26: 78-83.

[30] Malara NM, Leotta A, Sidoti A, Lio S, D'Angelo R, et al. (2006) Ageing, hormonal behaviour and cyclin D1 in ductal breast carcinomas. *Breast* 15: 81-89.

[31] Lerner LJ, Jordan VC (1990) Development of antiestrogens and their use in breast cancer: eighth Cain memorial award lecture. *Cancer Res* 50: 4177-4189.

[32] Weinberg OK, Marquez-Garban DC, Pietras RJ (2005) New approaches to reverse resistance to hormonal therapy in human breast cancer. *Drug Resist Updat* 8: 219-233.

[33] Kato S, Sato T, Watanabe T, Takemasa S, Masuhiro Y, et al. (2005) Function of nuclear sex hormone receptors in gene regulation. *Cancer Chemother Pharmacol* 56 Suppl 1: 4-9.

[34] Baykara M, Coskun U, Demirci U, Yildiz R, Benekli M, Cakir A and Buyukberber S (2010) Intracystic papillary carcinoma of the breast: one of the youngest patient in the literature. *Med Oncol* 27(4) 1427–8 DOI: 10.1007/s12032-009-9290-0.

[35] Umanah IN and Okpongette AS (2009) Intracystic papillary carcinoma of the breast in a 21-year old premenopausal Nigerian woman: a case report. *Rare Tumors* 1(2) e50 PMID: 21139929.

[36] Liberman L, Feng TL and Susnik B (2001) Case 35: intracystic papillary carcinoma with invasion. *Radiology* 219(3) 781–4 PMID: 11376269.

[37] . Dogan BE, Whitman GJ, Middleton LP et al. (2003) Intracystic papillary carcinoma of the breast. *AJR Am J Roentgenol* 181(1) 186 PMID: 12818855.

[38] Reefy S, Osman H, Chao C, Perry N and Mokbel K (2010) Surgical excision for B3 breast lesions diagnosed by vacuum-assisted core biopsy. *Anticancer Res* 30(6) 2287–90 PMID: 20651381.

[39] Yamamoto D, Ueda S, Senzaki H, Shoji T, Haijima H, Gondo H and Tanaka K (2001) New diagnostic approach to intracystic lesions of the breast by fiberoptic ductoscopy. *Anticancer Res* 21(6A) 4113–6.

[40] Mokbel K, Escobar PF and Matsunaga T (2005) Mammary ductoscopy: current status and future prospects. *Eur J Surg Oncol* 313–8 DOI: 10.1016/j.ejso.2004.10.004 PMID: 15642418.

[41] Tomonori K, Takayuki S, Tadahiko T, Hojo S, Akashi-Tanaka S, Murata Y. Clinical and pathological features of intracystic papillary carcinoma of the breast. *Surgery Today*. 2009; 39(1): 5–8.

[42] Benkaddour Y A, Hasnaoui S E, Fichtali K, Fakhir B, et al. Intracystic papillary carcinoma of the breast. Report of three cases and literature review. *Case Rep Obstetr Gynecol.* 2012, Article ID 979563.

[43] Kayahan M, Uzin M A, Ozkan O F, Gunes P, et al. Approach to papillary lesions of the breast (A Report of three cases). *The J Breast Health.* 2010; 6(4): 163-67.

[44] Rodriguez M C H, Secades A L, Angulo J M. Intracystic papillary carcinoma of the breast. *Radiographics.* 2010; 30:2021-2027.

[45] Esposito NN, Dabbs DJ, Bhargava R. Are encapsulated papillary carcinomas of the breast insitu or invasive? A basement membrane study of 27 cases. *American Soc Clin Pathol.* 2009; 131:228-242.

[46] Sara Al Reefy, Rashid Kameshki, Dhabya Al Sada, Abdullah Al Elewah, Arwa Al Awadhi, Kamil Al Awadhi. *ecancer* 2012;7:286-91.

[47] Noriko Yoshimura, Shigeru Murakami, Mayumi Kaneko, Akio Sakatani, Naoki Hirabayashi, and Wataru Takiyama, "Synchronous Bilateral Solid Papillary Carcinomas of the Breast," *Case Reports in Surgery* 2013;1155:8121-29.

[48] Gruber et al: Measurement of tumor size with mammography, sonography and magnetic resonance imaging as compared to histological tumor size in primary breast cancer. *BMC Cancer* 2013;13:328-36.

[49] Irina Anca Eremia, Maria Ciobanu, Tenea T, Maria Victoria Comanescu, Stefania Craitoiu. Invasive papillary carcinoma of the mammary gland:histopathologic and immunohistochemical aspects. *Rom J Morphol Embryol* 2012;53(3):811-815.

[50] Terzi A, Uner AH. An unusual case of invasive papillary carcinoma of the breast. *Indian J Pathol Microbiol* 2012;55:543-5.

[51] Bhosale SJ, Kshirsagar AY, Sulhyan SR, Jagtap SV, Nikam YP. *Case Rep Oncol* 2010;3:410-415.

[52] Mulligan AM and O'Malley FP (2007) Metastatic potential of encapsulated (intracystic) papillary carcinoma of the breast: a report of 2 cases with axillary lymph node micrometastases. *Int J Surg Pathol* 15(2) 143–7 DOI: 10.1177/1066896906299119 PMID: 17478767.

[53] Fayanju OM, Ritter J, Gillanders WE, Eberlein TJ, Dietz JR, Aft R and Margenthaler JA (2007) Therapeutic management of intracystic papillary carcinoma of the breast: the roles of radiation and endocrine therapy. *Am J Surg*194(4) 497–500,DOI: 10.1016/j.amjsurg.2007.06.016 PMID: 17826064.

[54] Mugler K, Marshal C, Hardesty L, Finlayson C and Singh M (2007) Intracystic papillary carcinoma of the breast: differential diagnosis and management. *Oncology* 21(7) 871–6 PMID: 17722745.

[55] Harris K, Faliakou E, Exon D, Nasiri N, Sacks NP and Gui GP (1999) Treatment and outcome of intracystic papillary carcinoma of the breast. *Br J Surg* 86 1274 DOI: 10.1046/j.1365-2168.1999.01254.x PMID: 10540131.

Chapter 12

Rare Tumors of Breast

A) Salivary Gland and Skin Adnexal-Type Tumors (Including Myoepithelial Tumors)

1) **Adenoid cystic carcinoma**
2) **Acinic cell carcinoma**
3) **Low grade adenosquamous carcinoma:-** is a well-differentiated tumor with dual glandular and squamous differentiation.
4) Glycogen rich (clear cell) carcinoma is composed of large clear cells, which are found to contain abundant glycogen [1, 2, 3].
5) Adenomyoepithelioma is a small (average diameter 1 cm), firm, well-circumscribed tumor microscopically composed of cells of polygonal shape and optically clear cytoplasm, arranged in nests that are sometimes centered by gland-forming epithelial cells [4].

B) Vascular Tumors and Tumorlike Lesions

1) Angiosarcoma (malignant hemangioendothelioma) of the breast characteristically occurs in young to middle-aged women [5]. Mammographically, it presents as a solitary mass that is usually uncalcified [6]. Grossly, the tumor is soft, spongy, and hemorrhagic.

Microscopically, the diagnostic areas are characterized by anastomosing vascular channels lined by atypical endothelial cells.

2) (Post-mastectomy; post-lymphedema) lymphangiosarcoma was a rare dreadful complication developing in the soft tissues of the upper extremity as a result of long-standing lymphedema following radical mastectomy or, exceptionally, segmental mastectomy [7].

C) Other Malignant Stromal Tumors

1) Stromal sarcoma is the generic term given to malignant breast tumors thought to arise from the specialized stroma of this organ but lacking an epithelial component with a phylloides pattern [8, 9]. Grossly, the tumors appear solid, grayish white, and homogeneous. Necrosis may be present. Microscopically, most of them have the features of fibrosarcoma; focal osseous metaplasia can occur. Infiltrative margins and severe atypia indicate a greater tendency for local recurrence and distant metastases [9].

D) Lymphoid Tumors. Malignant Lymphoma

- Burkit lymphoma
- Hodgkin lymphoma
- Anaplastic large cell lymphoma.
- Intravascular lymphoma.
- Myelocytic leukemia.

E) Breast Diseases in Males

Carcinoma:- In the United States, only 1% of all breast carcinomas occur in males, but in some Arab countries the incidence rises to nearly 10% [10, 11]. An increased incidence of breast carcinoma is seen in patients with Klinefelter syndrome [12]. Clinically, most breast carcinomas present in elderly individuals as breast nodules, with or without associated nipple abnormalities [13]. Nipple discharge in an adult male, especially if bloody, should arouse a strong suspicion of carcinoma. Skin involvement by fixation and Paget disease are much more common in males. Grossly, microscopically, and immunohistochemically, carcinomas of the male breast are very similar to those seen in females [10].

References

[1] Fisher ER, Tavares J, Bulatao IS, Sass R, Fisher Bcollaborating NSABP investigators: Glycogen-rich, clear cell breast cancer. With comments concerning other clear cell variants. *Hum Pathol* 1985; 16:1085-1090.

[2] Hayes MMM, Seidman JD, Ashton MA: Glycogen-rich clear cell carcinoma of the breast. A clinicopathologic study of 21 cases. *Am J Surg Pathol* 1995; 19:904-911.

[3] Hull MT, Warfel KA: Glycogen-rich clear cell carcinomas of the breast. A clinicopathologic and ultrastructural study. *Am J Surg Pathol* 1986; 10:553-559.

[4] Tavassoli FA: Myoepithelial lesions of the breast. Myoepitheliosis, adenomyoepithelioma, and myoepithelial carcinoma. *Am J Surg Pathol* 1991; 15:554-568.

[5] Vorburger SA, Xing Y, Hunt KK, Lakin GE, Benjamin RS, Feig BW, Pisters PW, Ballo MT, Chen L, Trent 3rd J, Burgess M, Patel S, Pollock RE, Cormier JN: Angiosarcoma of the breast. *Cancer* 2005; 104:2682-2688.

[6] Liberman L, Dershaw DD, Kaufman RJ, Rosen PP: Angiosarcoma of the breast. *Radiology* 1992; 183:649-654.

[7] Benda JA, Al-Jurf AS, Benson III AB: Angiosarcoma of the breast following segmental mastectomy complicated by lymphedema. *Am J clin Pathol* 1987; 87:651-655.

[8] Callery CD, Rosen PP, Kinne DW: Sarcoma of the breast. A study of 32 patients with reappraisal of classification and therapy. *Ann Surg* 1985; 201:527-532.

[9] Norris HJ, Taylor HB: Sarcomas and related mesenchymal tumors of the breast. *Cancer* 1968; 22:22-28.

[10] Donegan WL: Cancer of the breast in men. *CA Cancer J Clin* 1991; 41:339-354.

[11] El-Gazayerli M, Abdel-Aziz AS: On bilharziasis and male breast cancer in Egypt. A preliminary report and review of the literature. *Br J Cancer* 1963; 17:566-571.

[12] Sanchez AG, Villanueva AG, Redondo C: Lobular carcinoma of the breast in a patient with Klinefelter's syndrome. A case with bilateral, synchronous, histologically different breast tumors. *Cancer* 1986; 57:1181-1183.

[13] Cunha F, Andre S, Soares J: Morphology of male breast carcinoma in the evaluation of prognosis. *Pathol Res Pract* 1990; 186:745-750.

About the Authors

Dr. Sachin B. Ingle, MD
Department of Pathology,
Secretary Research & Development MIMSR Medical College,
Ambajogai Road, vishwanathpuram, Latur-Maharashtra 413531 India.
Telephone: +91-2382-227424 Fax: +91 -2382 -228939
dr.sachiningle@gmail.com

Dr. Priti Katkade
Resident Department of Pathology MIMSR Medical College
Latur, India

Dr. Kundan Chavan
Resident Department of Pathology MIMSR Medical College
Latur, India

Dr. Datta Girji
Professor and HOD Department of Pathology
Latur, India

Index

E

F

G

L

M

N

O

P

R

S